Mucocutaneous Lesions in DENTISTRY

Mucocutaneous Lesions in DENTISTRY

Vijay Kumar Biradar
PhD Scholar MDS
Department of Oral Pathology and Microbiology
Jaipur Dental College
Maharaj Vinayak Global University
Jaipur, Rajasthan, India

Forewords
Manohar Bhatt
Vela D Desai

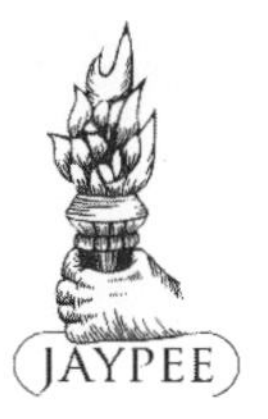

The Health Sciences Publisher

New Delhi | London | Philadelphia | Panama

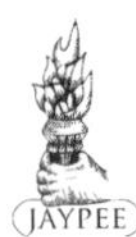

Jaypee Brothers Medical Publishers (P) Ltd

Headquarters

Jaypee Brothers Medical Publishers (P) Ltd
4838/24, Ansari Road, Daryaganj
New Delhi 110 002, India
Phone: +91-11-43574357
Fax: +91-11-43574314
Email: jaypee@jaypeebrothers.com

Overseas Offices

J.P. Medical Ltd
83 Victoria Street, London
SW1H 0HW (UK)
Phone: +44-2031708910
Fax: +44 (0)20 3008 6180
Email: info@jpmedpub.com

Jaypee Medical Inc
The Bourse
111 South Independence Mall East
Suite 835, Philadelphia, PA 19106, USA
Phone: +1 267-519-9789
Email: jpmed.us@gmail.com

Jaypee Brothers Medical Publishers (P) Ltd
Bhotahity, Kathmandu, Nepal
Phone: +977-9741283608
Email: kathmandu@jaypeebrothers.com

Jaypee-Highlights Medical Publishers Inc
City of Knowledge, Bld. 237, Clayton
Panama City, Panama
Phone: +1 507-301-0496
Fax: +1 507-301-0499
Email: cservice@jphmedical.com

Jaypee Brothers Medical Publishers (P) Ltd
17/1-B Babar Road, Block-B, Shaymali
Mohammadpur, Dhaka-1207
Bangladesh
Mobile: +08801912003485
Email: jaypeedhaka@gmail.com

Website: www.jaypeebrothers.com
Website: www.jaypeedigital.com

Inquiries for bulk sales may be solicited at: jaypee@jaypeebrothers.com

Mucocutaneous Lesions in Dentistry

First Edition: **2016**

ISBN 978-93-5250-040-6

Printed at Rajkamal Electric Press, Plot No. 2, Phase-IV, Kundli, Haryana.

Foreword

Many books about diseases of the oral mucosa, oral manifestations of acquired immunodeficiency syndrome (AIDS), and other diseases of the oral cavity have been published in recent years. Several excellent textbooks of oral pathology have also appeared. In this comprehensive book, *Mucocutaneous Lesions in Dentistry*, the author has arranged the etiological, clinical and histopathological information of mucocutaneous lesions systematically. This combination will permit a successful search for the correct definitive diagnosis. The subject is written and presented in a simple and lucid style, which makes it easy to understand and interesting to read. Appropriate subject-oriented photographs, tables and illustrations are invaluable contribution. I have no doubt that the simplicity of the text and its exceptional clarity will be much appreciated by the readers. He has also taken care to reduce redundancy within the text whenever possible.

Manohar Bhatt MDS
Principal
Jaipur Dental College
Maharaj Vinayak Global University
Jaipur, Rajasthan, India

Foreword

It is a great pleasure for me to write foreword for the book *Mucocutaneous Lesions in Dentistry*. This subject is very important and is often neglected by dental clinicians. This book is enriched with good quality photographs. The language of this book is very simple and easy to understand. This book covers all the topics related to mucocutaneous lesions in dentistry. The author has to be congratulated for further improving on the innovative excellent format. The book has been designed in such a way that the students, teachers, research scholars and practitoners will get full and clear mental picture of the subject.

I wish the author and this book all success.

Vela D Desai MDS
Professor and Head
Department of Oral Medicine and Radiology
Jaipur Dental College
Jaipur, Rajasthan, India

Preface

It is axiomatic in all branches of medicine that treatment is based on accurate diagnosis. The treatment of mucocutaneous lesions is no exception to this axiom. There are many diseases that affect the orofacial region of the body. Of these, many appear as oral manifestations of dermatologic diseases of the body, while others are purely local oral diseases. Some of these diseases, if not treated, may complicate various tissues of the body. This book, *Mucocutaneous Lesions in Dentistry*, deals with classification, etiopathogenesis, clinical features, histopathological features, diagnosis, differential diagnosis, treatment and prognosis of each mucocutaneous lesion. This is not a textbook, but a field guide to mucocutaneous diagnosis.

There had been a long-standing demand from BDS and MDS students for a book of "Oral Manifestations of Dermatologic Lesions" which would help them in providing a deductive method of approach in mucocutaneous diagnosis.

This book is structured to cover the essential aspects of mucocutaneous lesions for undergraduate and postgraduate students. It contains 20 chapters with clinical and histopathological photographs and references.

Vijay Kumar Biradar

Acknowledgments

First and foremost I bow in gratitude to the Almighty God for His blessings.

I acknowledge all the help provided by Managing Director, Dr Vikas Jeph and Principal, Dr Manohar Bhatt, Jaipur Dental College, Maharaja Vinayak Global University, Jaipur, Rajasthan, India towards bringing out this book.

I am grateful to all my teachers Dr R Rajendran, Dr VT Beena and Dr Heera R, who have been a constant source of inspiration during my postgraduation in Government Dental College, Thiruvananthapuram, Kerala, India.

I am extremely thankful to Dr Shrinivas Vanaki, Principal and Head, Department of Oral Pathology, PMNM Dental College and Hospital, Bagalkote, Karnataka, India, for his constant support and encouragement.

I am also indebted to the following people, for their timely and much needed help in writing this book, viz. Dr Madhusudan Astekar, Dr Anuja Holani, Dr Mangala Meti, Dr Veena Kalburgi, Dr Manoj Jain, Dr Rupeesh, Dr Nilesh Pardhe, Dr Kunal and Manish.

This book would not have been accomplished if much needed help would not have come from Dr Surekha Angadi.

A special gratitude is offered to my family for their patience and support.

I finally acknowledge my sincere thanks to Shri Jitendar P Vij (Group Chairman), Mr Ankit Vij (Group President), Mr Tarun Duneja (Director-Publishing) of M/s Jaypee Brothers Medical Publishers (P) Ltd, New Delhi, India, and Mr Ramesh Krishnacharya and Ms Shilpi Dutta (staff of Kolkata branch), for their acceptance and endeavor to bring this text in an excellent book form.

Contents

Chapter 1: Introduction and Classification **1–8**
- Dermatologic lesions 1
- Primary lesions 2
- Secondary skin lesions 4
- Vascular lesions 6
- Classification of skin diseases 7

Chapter 2: Hereditary Ectodermal Dysplasia **9–15**
- Pathogenesis 9
- Classification 11
- Clinical features 12
- Oral manifestations 13
- Histopathologic features 14
- Diagnosis 14
- Differential diagnosis 15
- Treatment 15
- Prognosis 15

Chapter 3: Hypersensitivity Reactions **16–23**

Chapter 4: Oral Lichen Planus **24–32**
- Etiology and pathogenesis 24
- Clinical features 25
- Oral manifestations 27
- Classification 28
- Differential diagnosis 30
- Management 30

Chapter 5: Systemic Sclerosis **33–38**
- Pathogenesis 33
- Clinical features 34
- Classification 34
- Oral manifestations 36
- Histologic features 37
- Diagnosis 38
- Treatment 38

Chapter 6: CREST Syndrome (Acrosclerosis) **39–41**
- Clinical features 39
- Diagnosis 40
- Histologic features 41
- Treatment and prognosis 41

Chapter 7: Psoriasis **42–44**
- Etiopathogenesis 42
- Clinical features 42
- Oral manifestations 43

- Histologic features 43
- Differential diagnosis 44
- Treatment 44
- Prognosis 44

Chapter 8: Pemphigus **45–54**
- Epithelial biology 45
- Pemphigus and variants 46
- Pemphigus vulgaris 48
- Possible etiologic factors 50
- Clinical features 51
- Histologic features 51
- Treatment and prognosis 53

Chapter 9: Paraneoplastic Pemphigus **55–58**
- Clinical features 56
- Pathogenesis 57
- Diagnostic criteria 57
- Treatment 58

Chapter 10: Pemphigoid and Other Basement Membrane Diseases **59–68**
- Classification of pemphigoid group of diseases 60
- Epithelial biology 60
- Mucous membrane pemphigoid 62
- Direct immunofluorescence (DIF) 65

Chapter 11: Erythema Multiforme **69–82**
- Toxic epidermal necrolysis (Lyell's syndrome) 80
- Drug-related erythema multiforme 81
- Drug-related toxic epidermal necrolysis 82

Chapter 12: Lupus Erythematosus **83–94**
- Pathogenesis 83
- Clinical features 84
- Mucocutaneous disease 86
- Histopathology 92

Chapter 13: Epidermolysis Bullosa **95–101**
- Pathogenesis 95
- Epidermolysis bullosa simplex 97
- Junctional epidermolysis bullosa 98
- Epidermolysis bullosa dystrophic, dominant 98
- Epidermolysis bullosa dystrophic, recessive 99

Chapter 14: Darier's Disease **102–108**
- Pathogenesis 102
- Clinical features 104
- Diagnosis 106
- Treatment 107

Chapter 15: Dyskeratosis Congenita **109–113**
- Pathogenesis 109
- Clinical features 109
- Oral manifestations 110
- Histologic findings 112
- Treatment 113

Chapter 16: White Sponge Nevus **114–118**
- Pathogenesis 114
- Clinical features and oral manifestations 115
- Histologic features 116
- Treatment 117

Chapter 17: Warty Dyskeratosis **119–120**
- Clinical features 119
- Histologic features 119
- Treatment and prognosis 119

Chapter 18: Cowden Syndrome **121–126**
- Pathogenesis 121
- Clinical features 121
- Differential diagnosis 126
- Treatment 126

Chapter 19: Peutz-Jeghers Syndrome **127–130**
- Pathogenesis 127
- Clinical features 128
- Diagnosis 129
- Differential diagnosis 129
- Treatment and prognosis 130

Chapter 20: Hereditary Benign Intraepithelial Dyskeratosis **131–133**
- Clinical presentation 131
- Treatment 133

Index *135–136*

CHAPTER 1

Introduction and Classification

DERMATOLOGIC LESIONS

Introduction

Dermatologic diagnosis is based up on systematic approach which includes history, physical examination and diagnostic tests.

There are some relevant aspects that must be asked in the history:

- Age.
- Breed.
- Sex.
- Occupation (work environment).
- Geographic location.
- Previous skin diseases.
- Associated symptoms (itching, pain, etc.).
- Therapy used and response.
- Exacerbation of the lesions by the sun or irritating substances exposure.
- Similar cases in family.

In the physical examination, the appearance of the lesion is an important feature to be considered, that is why a necessary careful approach and detailed examination must proceed as follows:

Dermatology classifies lesions primarily by their visual appearance and texture. Lesions are divided into two general categories, primary and secondary. Primary lesions are those that are directly associated with the disease process and usually appear early in the course of the disease. Those appearing later are called secondary lesions and may be a result of the ongoing disease process and changes to the primary lesions.

A morphological classification of dermatological lesions is most helpful to the identification of the diseases present.

Primary lesions	*Secondary lesions*
• Macules	• Scale
• Papules	• Crust
• Plaque	• Fissure
• Nodules	• Scar
• Vesicles	• Excoriation
• Bulla	• Lichenification
• Wheals	• Erosion
• Pustules	• Atrophy
• Cysts	• Ulcer
• Purpura	
• Petechiae	
• Ecchymoses	
• Telangiectasia	

PRIMARY LESIONS

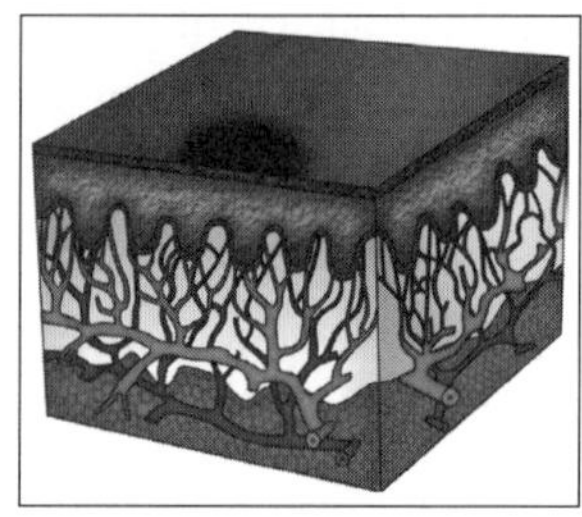

Macule: Well-circumscribed, flat lesions that are noticeable because of their change from normal skin color. They may be red due to the presence of vascular lesions or due to inflammation, or pigmented due to the presence of melanin, hemosiderin, and drugs.

E.g.

- Ephelis or freckle
- Vitiligo
- Tinea versicolor.

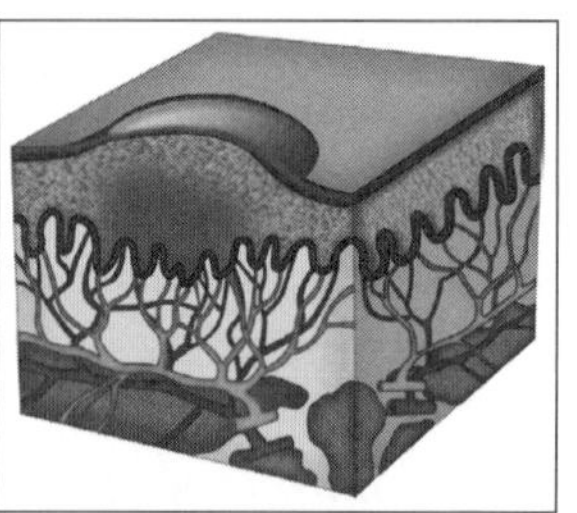

Papule: Elevated, solid and circumscribed lesion, usually 1 cm or less in diameter.

E.g.

- Hyperkeratotic: Warts, seborrheic keratoses
- Purple: Drug eruptions, Kaposi's sarcoma
- Red: Erythema multiforme, scabies.

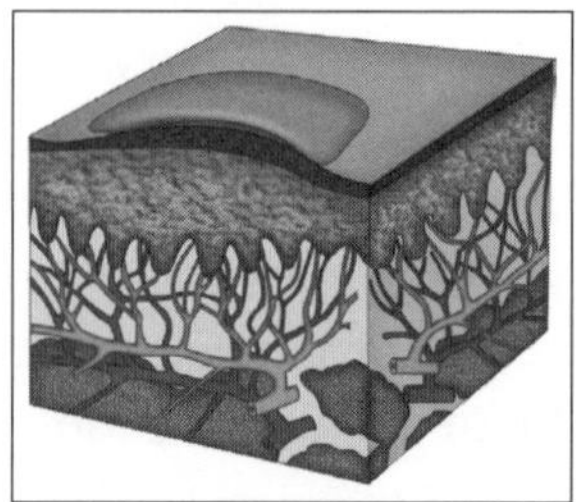

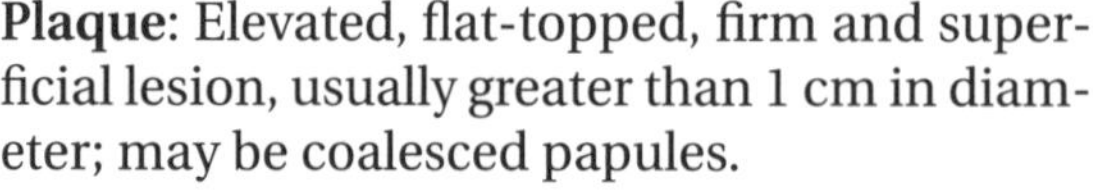

Plaque: Elevated, flat-topped, firm and superficial lesion, usually greater than 1 cm in diameter; may be coalesced papules.

E.g.

- Psoriasis
- Eczematous dermatitis.

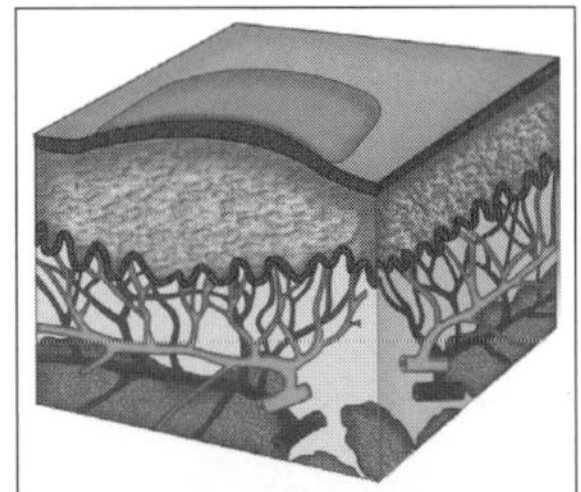

Wheal: Transient, solid, itchy, raised area of cutaneous edema with irregular shape, different diameter and variable blanching and erythema.

E.g.

- Urticaria
- Insect bites.

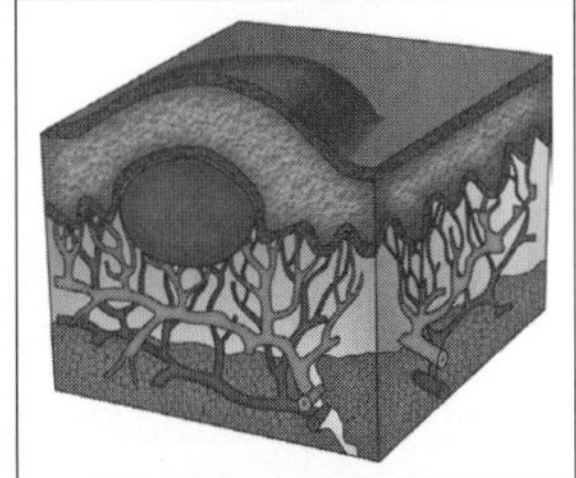

Nodule: Solid raised, circumscribed, firm lesion; variable diameter (usually 1–3 cm); deeper in dermis than papule. It can be seen in gross inspection or only on palpation.

E.g.

- Lipoma
- Erythema nodosum.

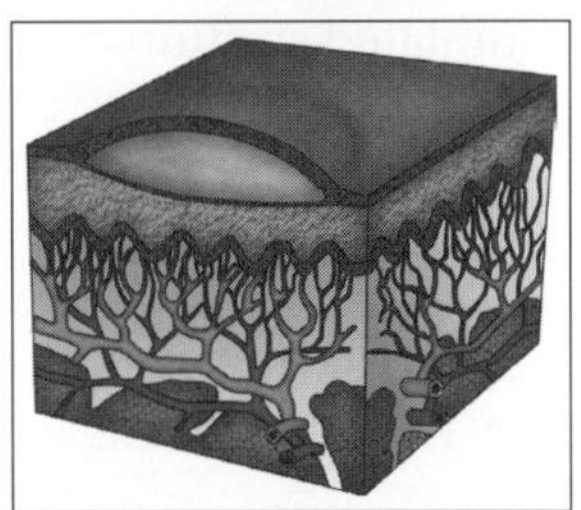

Vesicle: Elevated, thin-walled lesion, filled with serous (clear) fluid, less than 1 cm in diameter.

E.g.

- Herpes simplex
- Varicella-Herpes zoster
- Dermatitis herpetiformis.

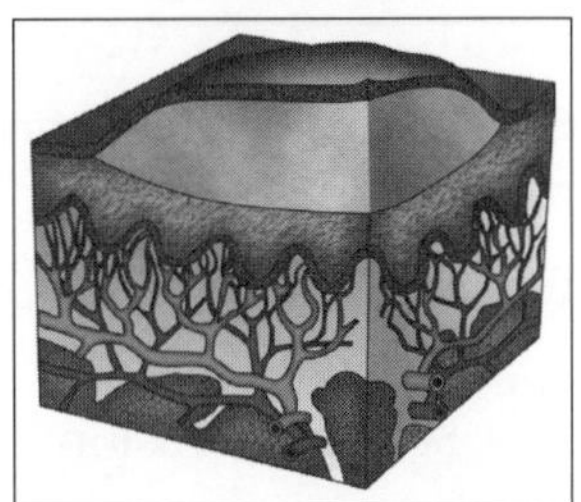

Bulla: Elevated lesion filled with clear fluid, greater than 1 cm in diameter.

E.g.

- Pemphigus
- Pemphigoid
- Drug eruptions
- Stevens-Johnson syndrome
- Blister.

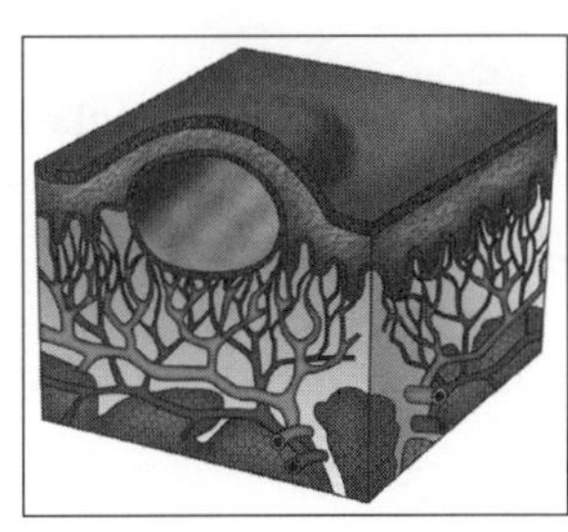

Cyst: Elevated and encapsulated lesion filled with semisolid, liquid or gaseous content.

E.g.

- Sebaceous cyst
- Cystic acne.

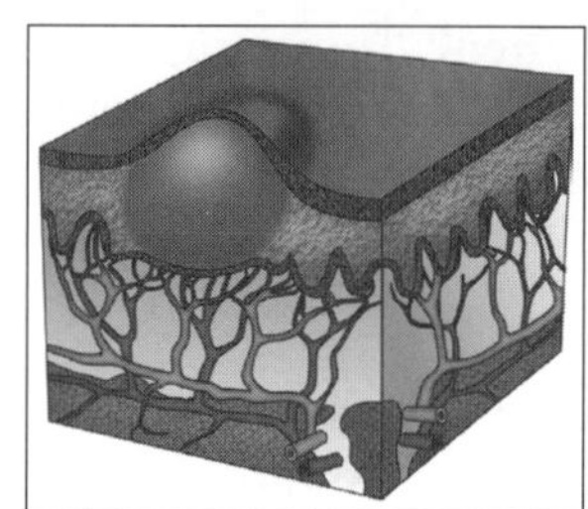

Pustule: Elevated lesion filled with purulent fluid. The presence of the pustule does not necessarily signify the existence of an infection.

E.g.

- Acne vulgaris
- Impetigo
- Variola
- Folliculitis
- Candidiasis.

SECONDARY SKIN LESIONS

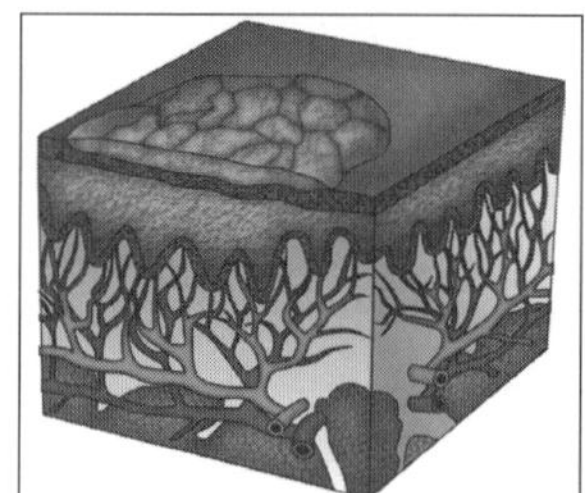

Scale: Flaky exfoliation, a plate-like excrescence of varied size, usually composed of accumulated stratum corneum.

E.g.

- Psoriasis
- Dermatitis
- Tinea versicolor
- Pityriasis rosea.

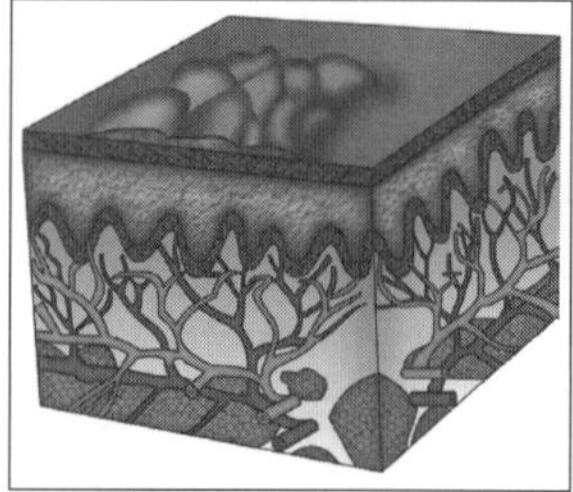

Crust (scab): A solid consolidation of dried serum, blood, pus.

E.g.

- Eczema
- Scab on abrasion.

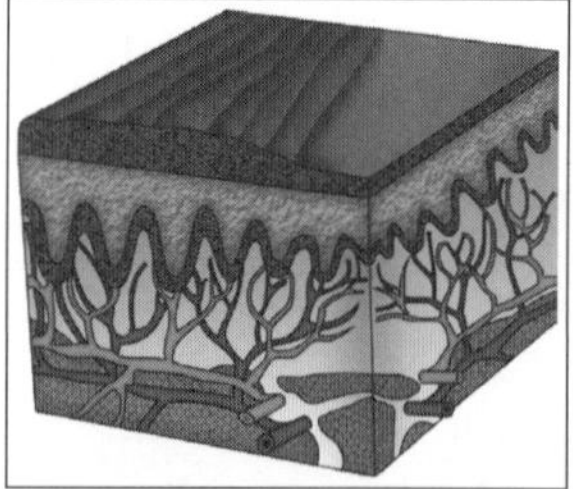

Lichenification: Thickened and rough epidermis with accentuation of skin markings.

E.g.

- Chronic contact eczema.

Scar: Fibrous tissue secondary to dermis injury. It may be pink, red or white; atrophic or hypertrophic (keloid).

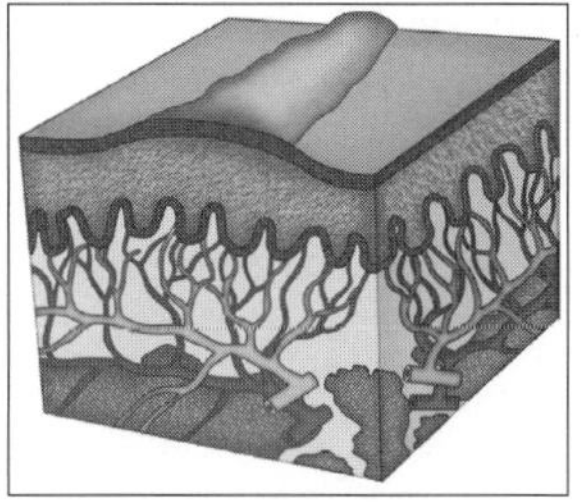

E.g.

- Healed wound.

Excoriation: Loss of epidermis caused by a traumatic lesion causing a linear area.

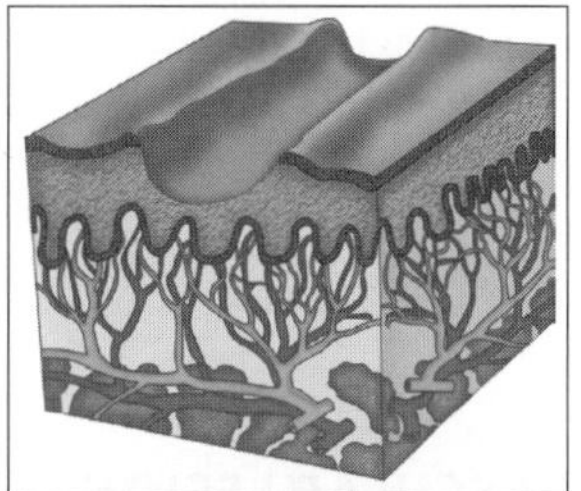

E.g.

- Deep scratch
- Abrasion.

Fissure: A linear and small split or crack in the epidermis and dermis.

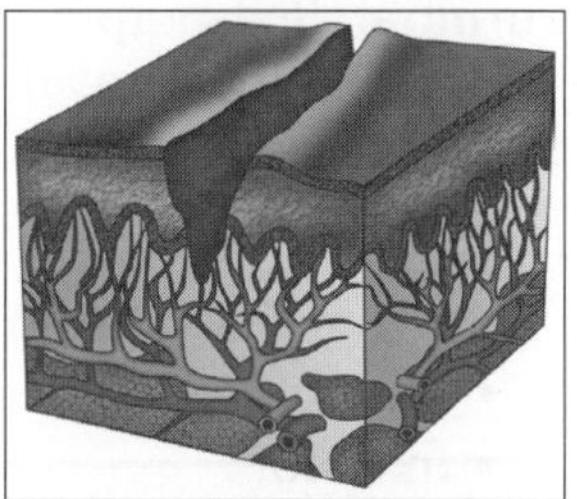

E.g.

- Cheilosis.

Erosion: Discontinuity of the skin with loss of part or all epidermis, usually follows rupture of vesicle or bulla.

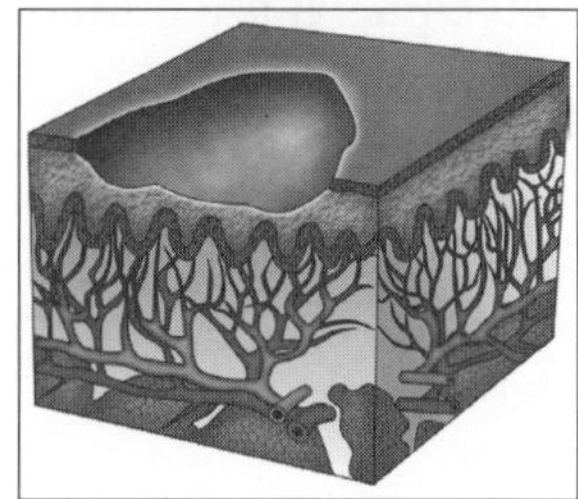

E.g.

- Varicella (following rupture)
- Variola (following rupture).

Ulceration: Discontinuity of the skin with loss of epidermis; and sometimes hipodermis. Usually heals with scaring.

E.g.

- Decubitus
- Herpes simplex
- Syphilis (chancre).

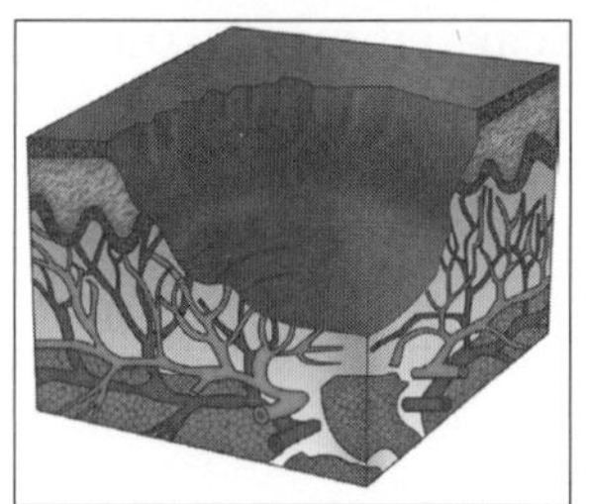

Ulcers: Ulceration without tendency of healing (scaring).

E.g.

- Stasis ulcers.

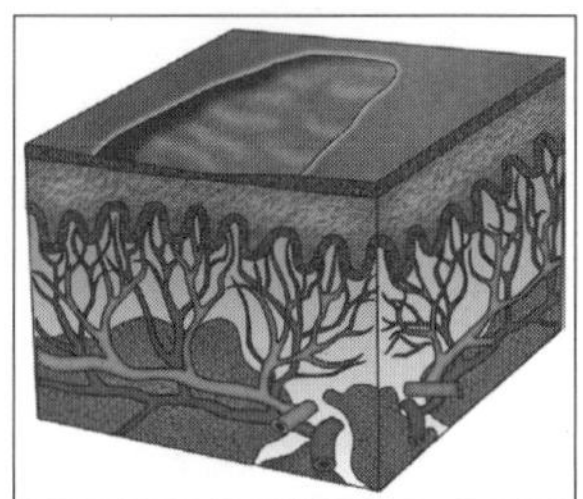

Atrophy: Reduction of skin thickening ocurring at any skin layer.

E.g.

- Striae
- Aged skin.

VASCULAR LESIONS

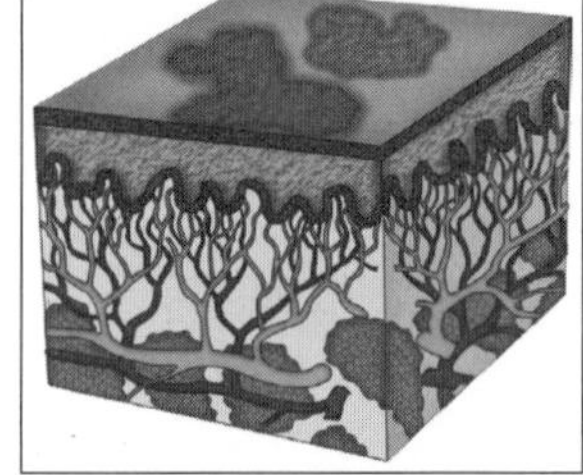

Purpura: Red-purple nonblanching colored lesion due to extravation of blood into the tissue.

E.g.

- Henoch-Schönlein purpura
- Thrombocytopenic purpura
- Infection.

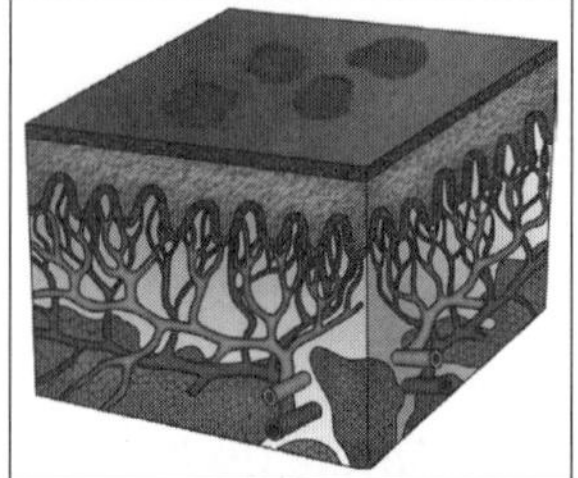

Petechiae: It is a punctiform purpura.

E.g.

- Vasculitis
- Infection.

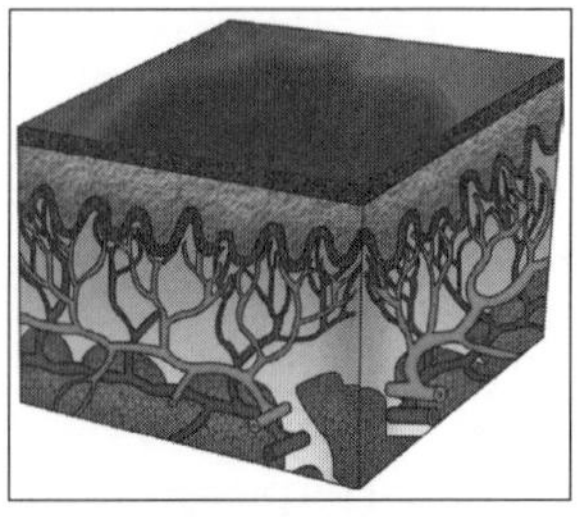

Ecchymoses: Purpura greater than 1 cm in diameter.

E.g.

- Trauma
- Vasculitis.

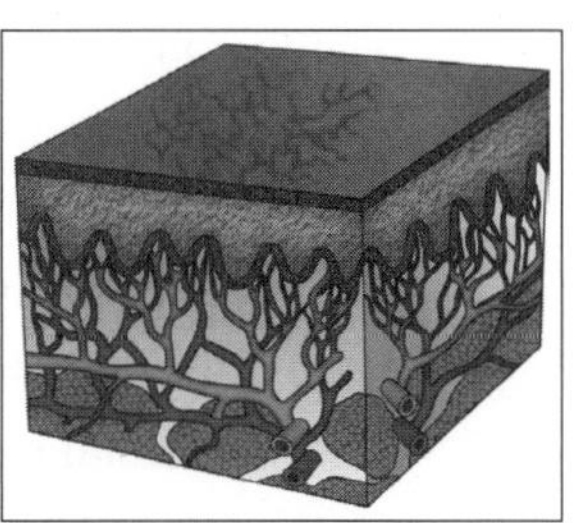

Telangiectasia: Permanent dilated superficial blood vessels.

E.g.

- Telangiectasia in liver disease
- Telangiectasia in pregnancy
- Telangiectasia in breast cancer
- Telangiectasia in lupus erythematosus, systemic or discoid.

CLASSIFICATION OF SKIN DISEASES

Dermatologic lesions may be classified as immune mediated diseases, vesiculobullous diseases, and diseases that are genetically transmitted.

Andrews and Regezi classification

I. Congenital ectodermal defects
   1. Hypohidrotic ectodermal dysplasia (Anhidrotic ectodermal dysplasia)
   2. Hidrotic ectodermal dysplasia (Clouston syndrome)

II. Immune-mediated diseases (Papules and plaques)
   1. Lichen planus
      i. Linear lichen planus (Zosteriform lichen planus)
      ii. Annular lichen planus
      iii. Hypertrophic lichen planus (Lichen planus verrucosus)
      iv. Ulcerative lichen planus
      v. Bullous lichen planus
      vi. Follicular lichen planus
      vii. Drug-induced lichen planus
   2. Reiter's syndrome
   3. Graft versus host disease
   4. Systemic sclerosis
   5. CREST syndrome
   6. Papulosquamous dermatoses
   7. Psoriasis
   8. Pityriasis rosea.

III. Chronic blistering dermatoses
   1. Pemphigus (Vesicles bulla/pustules)
      i. Pemphigus vulgaris

ii. Pemphigus vegetans
iii. Pemphigus foliaceus
iv. Brazilian pemphigus
v. Pemphigus erythematosus
2. Paraneoplastic pemphigus
3. Cicatricial pemphigoid
4. Epidermolysis bullosa acquisita
5. Dermatitis herpetiformis.

IV. Vesicles/bullae/pustules

Erythema and Urticaria

1. Erythema multiforme
2. Erythema migrans
3. Drug-induced bullous erythema multiforme
(Stevens-Johnsons syndrome)
Toxic epidermal necrolysis
Annular urticarial reactions

V. Endocrine diseases

1. Acanthosis nigricans

VI. Connective tissue diseases

1. Lupus erythematosus
(Systemic + discoid) lupus erythematosus

VII. Some genodermatosis and acquired syndromes

1. Epidermolysis bullosa
2. Pachyonychia congenita
3. Darier's disease
4. Hailey-Hailey disease
5. Incontinentia pigmenti
6. Dyskeratosis congenita
7. Porokeratosis.
(Plaque type porokeratosis Mibelli)

VIII Epidermal nevi

1. White sponge nevus

IX Dermatoses resulting from physical factors

1. Solar elastosis

X Abnormalities of dermal connective tissue

1. Ehlers-Danlos syndrome.

CHAPTER

2

Hereditary Ectodermal Dysplasia

INTRODUCTION

Ectodermal dysplasias (EDs) are a large group of nosologically complex diseases. More than 170 different pathological clinical conditions have been recognized and defined as EDs. EDs form part of a wide range of syndromes presenting abnormal development of two or more tissues derived from the ectoderm. They are nonprogressive, diffuse, congenital genodermatoses, characterized by a lack or scarcity of hair, teeth, nails and eccrine sweat glands, to which can be added defects in the external morphology (nose, outer ears, and lips), disorders of the CNS; alterations of the eyes; anomalies in the oronasal mucosa and in melanocytes.

It was first described by Thurnam in 1848 and was coined by Weech in 1929. In 1875, Charles Darwin documented it amongst a Hindu family of *Scinde* where 10 men in the course of 4 generations were affected. It is remarkable that no instance has occurred of a daughter being affected.

PATHOGENESIS

Recently, several gene defects causing ectodermal dysplasia syndromes have been characterized (Table 2.1). One of the most recently cloned gene behind these syndromes is *PVRL1* that encodes a cell-cell adhesion molecule nectin 1. Mutations of PVRL1 gene are behind cleft lip/palate, ectodermal dysplasia syndrome. These patients have sparse eyebrows and eyelashes, sparse hair and hypodontia. In addition, the patients have cleft lip/palate, syndactyly of fingers and toes and onychodysplasia.

Table 2.1 Mutated genes in human ectodermal dysplasia syndromes

Gene	*Types of protein*	*Ectodermal dysplasia*	*References*
Eda	TNF	X-linked HED	Kere, et al. 1996 Bayes, et al. 1998
Edar	TNFR	Autosomal recessive HED Autosomal dominant HED	Monreal, et al. 1999

Contd...

Contd...

Gene	*Types of protein*	*Ectodermal dysplasia*	*References*
Edaradd	DD containing adaptor protein	Autosomal recessive HED	Headon and Overbeek, 2001
IκBα	Inhibitor of NκBα	EDA-ID	Courtois, et al. 2003
IKKγ	Subunit of IKK	Incontinentia pigmenti	Smahi, et al. 2000
		OL-EDA-ID	
		HED-ID	Döffinger, et al. 2001 Zonana, et al. 2000
Plako-philin 1	Cytoplasmic desmosomal plaque protein	Ectodermal dysplasia/ skin fragility syndrome	McGrath, et al. 1997
Pvrl1	Adherens junction protein	ED4 (Margarita Island Type)	Suzuki, et al. 2000
Connexin 30	Gap junction component	Clouston syndrome	Lamartine, et al. 2000
P63	Transcription factor	EEC	Celli, et al. 1999
		LMS	van Bokhoeven, et al. 2001
		SHFM	Ianakiev, et al. 2000
		AEC	McGrath, et al. 2001
		ADULT	Amiel, et al. 2003
		RHS	Kantaputra, et al. 2003
Keratins 6A, 6B Keratins 16, 17	Structural filamentous proteins	Pachyonychia congenita I, II	Bowden, et al. 1995 Mc Lean, et al. 1995 Smith, et al. 1998

Transmission of hypohidrotic ectodermal dysplasia is, in general, X-linked (females carry the responsible gene, and males suffer from the disease, although the carrying mothers usually bear some typical characteristic feature of the disease) and at times in autosomal recessive form. Mosaic expression is rare. Currently, hypohidrotic ectodermal dysplasia is related with a mutation of the protein ectodysplasin-A, related with the EDA gene in the q12–q13 locus of the X chromosome (consisting of 12 exons, 8 of which are responsible for encoding the EDA-A1 transmembrane protein which is related with ectodermal growth). Mutations in one or various genes, including EDA, EDAR (EDA receptor) and NEMO (NF-kB essential modulator: encodes the NEMO protein, regulator of NF-kB transcription factor activity that intervenes in the control of stratified epithelial growth, allowing the cells to respond to external stimuli, etc.) are associated with hypohidrotic ectodermal dysplasia, with or without immunodeficiency.

Mutations in NEMO that suppress the protein synthesis (amorphic mutations) cause incontinentia pigmenti, however, the hypomorphic mutations in NEMO that do not eliminate its entire function cause ectodermic dysplasias and immunodeficiency in man.

CLASSIFICATION

Ectodermal dysplasia is a relatively rare disorder, with a frequency varying between 1:10,000 and 1:100,000 live births, and is more frequent in males. The majority of cases follow the autosomal-recessive mode of inheritance, but it can also be autosomal-dominant or X-linked.

The most frequently observed types of ectodermic dysplasia are (Table 2.2):

- Hypohidrotic-anhidrotic
- Hidrotic.

The hypohidrotic-anhidrotic type, or Christ-Siemens-Touraine syndrome was first described in 1848 by Thurman, and is characterized by the triad of hypotrichosis (skin, hair and nail anomalies), either hypodontia or anodontia, and hypohidrosis (partial or total absence of eccrine sweat glands) and other features such as frontal bossing, saddle-shaped nose, everted lips, etc. Felsher in 1944 changed the adjective anhydrotic to hypohydrotic because the persons with hypohydrotic form are not truly devoid of all sweat glands.

The hidrotic type was first defined in 1929 by Clouston, and is distinguished by hypotrichosis, ungual dystrophy and hyperkeratosis of the palms and soles.

Numerous combinations of clinical alterations can present in ectodermal dysplasia, observing diverse syndromes and upto 154 different types of ectodermal dysplasias and 11 subgroups, labeled from 1 to 4 according to whether they affect the hair, teeth, nails or sweat glands.

A definitive classification of ED was difficult to formulate since many of the syndrome that involve ED have overlapping features. A simple attempt made by Nelson included 5 categories, namely

- Hypohidrotic (Anhidrotic)
- Hidrotic (Clouston syndrome)
- EEC (Ectodactyly ectodermal dysplasia) syndrome
- Rapp-Hodgkin syndrome
- Robinson disease.

While Lamartine has classified the ED genes into 4 major functional subgroups:

- Cell communication and signaling
- Cell adhesion
- Transcription regulation
- Development.

In 2001, Priolo and Lagana proposed a new classification based on the latest molecular genetic data and corresponding clinical findings. Under this new classification, EDs are subdivided into 2 groups:

- Group I: It includes disorders involving a defect in developmental regulation and in epithelial-mesenchymal interaction.
- Group II: It includes disorders in which a structural protein defect has been found or can be inferred from specific clinical features.

CLINICAL FEATURES[1, 3, 4]

It is typically inherited as a cross-linked recessive trait so that the frequency and severity of the condition is more pronounced in males than in females. Furthermore, it was redefined by Freire-Maia as a developmental defect which at embryonic level affects the ectoderm and therefore, the tissues and structures derived from it. Thus, it affects the development of keratinocytes and cause aberrations in the hair, sebaceous glands, eccrine and apocrine glands, nails, teeth, lenses and conjunctiva of the eyes, anterior pituitary gland, nipples and the ears.

The disorder might occur during the first trimester of pregnancy. If it is severe, it appears before the 6th week of embryonic life and consequently the dentition will be affected. After 8th week other ectodermal structure may be affected.

Affected individuals typically display heat intolerance because of a reduced number of sweat glands. Sometimes, the diagnosis is made during infancy because the baby appears to have a fever of undetermined origin, however, the infant simply cannot regulate body temperature appropriately because of the decreased number of sweat glands. Uncommonly, death results from the markedly elevated body temperature. Sometimes, a diagnostic aid, a special impression can be made of the patient's fingertips and then examined microscopically to count the density of the sweat glands. Such findings should be interpreted in conjunction with appropriate age-matched controls.

Other signs of this disorder include fine, sparse blonde hair, including a reduced density of eyebrow and eyelash hair (Fig. 2.1).

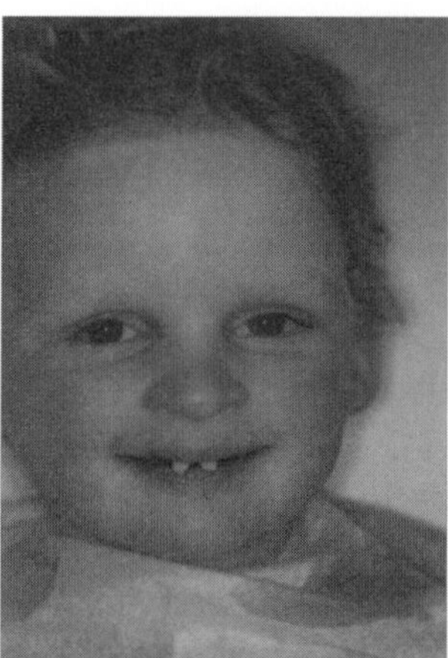

Fig. 2.1: Reduced density of eyebrow and eyelash hair

The periocular skin may show a fine wrinkling with hyperpigmentation, and midface hypoplasia is frequently observed, often resulting in protuberant lips. Because the salivary glands are ectodermally derived, patients may exhibit varying degrees of xerostomia. The nails may also appear dystrophic and brittle.

ORAL MANIFESTATIONS

The teeth are usually markedly reduced in number (oligodontia or hypodontia), and their crown shapes are characteristically abnormal (Fig. 2.2). The incisor crowns usually appear tapered, conical, or pointed, and the molar crowns are reduced in diameter (Fig. 2.3). Complete lack of tooth development (anodontia) has also been reported, but this appears to be uncommon.

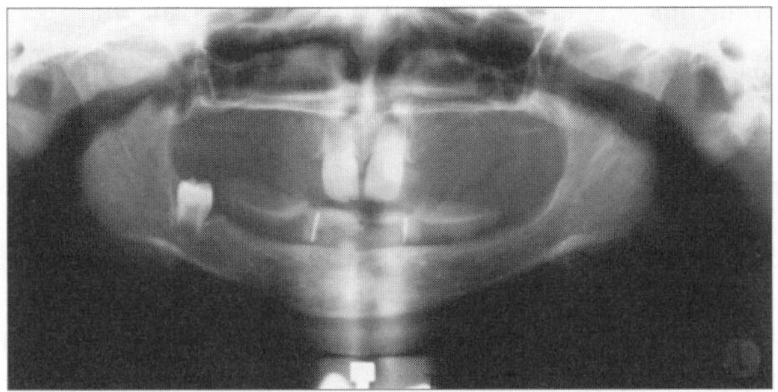

Fig. 2.2: Severe hypodontia in both the mandible and the maxilla

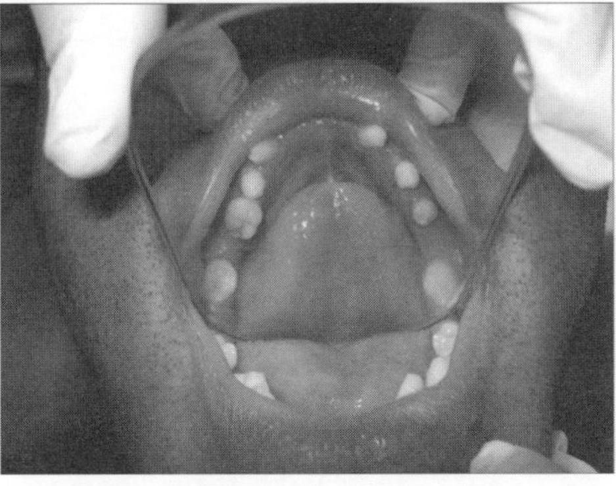

Fig. 2.3: Incisor and molar crowns are tapered, and conical

Female patients may show partial expression of the abnormal gene; that is, their teeth may be reduced in number or may have mild structural changes. This incomplete presentation can be explained by the Lyon hypothesis, with half of the female patient's X chromosomes expressing the normal gene and the other half expressing the defective gene.

Table 2.2: Differences between hidrotic and hypohidrotic EDs

	Hidrotic	*Hypohidrotic*
Mode of inheritance	Most often autosomal dominant	Most often autosomal recessive
Scalp hair	Soft, dawny, color is darker	Fine in texture, fair and short
	Hidrotic	*Hypohidrotic*
Teeth	Anodontia to hypodontia	Anodontia to hypodontia
Lips	No abnormality	Protruding
Sweat glands	Active	Reduced to absent
Nasal bridge	No flattening	Underdeveloped
Nails	Dystrophic nails	No abnormality
Eyebrows/eyelashes	Frequently absent	Absent
Pubic/axillary hairs	Scanty/absent	Variably affected

HISTOPATHOLOGIC FEATURES

Histopathologic examination of the skin from a patient with hypohidrotic ectodermal dysplasia shows a decreased number of sweat glands and hair follicles (Fig. 2.4). The adnexal structures that are present are hypoplastic and malformed.

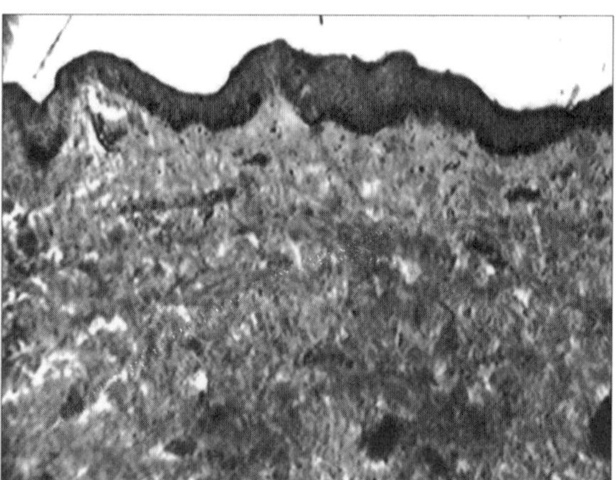

Fig. 2.4: Stratified squamous keratinized epithelium showing absence of sweat glands and hair follicle

DIAGNOSIS

The diagnosis of patients with ectodermal dysplasia is based fundamentally on the clinical history (ungula dystrophy, hypotrichosis, anodontia, oligodontia, hypodontia); on a skin biopsy in cases of changes in sweating (reduction in pilosebaceous units and sweat glands); hair study showing thin, fine hair; panoramic radiography (clearly showing dental dysmorphia and agenesis); molecular genetic analysis (studying genetic mutation, genetic locus, EDA, EDAR, NEMO, etc.).

DIFFERENTIAL DIAGNOSIS

The differential diagnosis of ectodermal dysplasias should be made against pathologies such as—congenital syphilis, familial simple anhidrosis, aplasia cutis congenita, dyskeratosis congenita, fever of unknown origin, progeroid syndromes such as Werner syndrome or Rothmund-Thomson syndrome, pachyonychia congenita, recurrent infant pneumonia, etc.

TREATMENT[2]

Management of hypohidrotic ectodermal dysplasia warrants genetic counseling for the parents and patient. The dental problems are best managed by prosthetic replacement of the dentition with complete dentures, overdentures, or fixed appliances, depending on the number and location of the remaining teeth. With careful site selection, endosseous dental implants may be considered for facilitating prosthetic management of patients older than 5 years of age.

PROGNOSIS

The prognosis is usually good, except in cases with hypo or anhidrosis, where mortality rates can reach 30% in first infancy, due fundamentally to respiratory infections resulting from the absence of mucosal glands in the respiratory system.

REFERENCES

1. Sharmal J, Mamatha GP. Hereditary ectodermal dysplasia: Diagnostic dilemmas. Rev Clín Pesq Odontol. Curitiba, 2008;4(1):35–40.
2. Adolfo Pipa Vallejo, Elena López- Arranz Monje. Treatment with removable prosthesis in hypohidrotic ectodermal dysplasia. A clinical case. Med Oral Patol Oral Cir Bucal 2008 1;13(2):E119–23.
3. Bai-Yao Wu, Wei-Ming Wang. Sporadic anhidrotic ectodermal dysplasia associated with vitiligo. J Med Sci 2004;24(3):149–52.
4. Neville, Damm, Allen, Bouquot. Oral and Maxillofacial Pathology; 2nd ed, Dermatologic diseases.

CHAPTER 3

Hypersensitivity Reactions

INTRODUCTION

Type I. Immediate or Anaphylactic Hypersensitivity

Immediate or anaphylactic hypersensitivity is mediated by IgE antibodies, which are bound to mast cells and basophils. When the allergen reacts with them, mediators, which are preformed and stored within the cell's granules, are released (degranulation).The reaction is immediate; the clinical effect is usually severe and dependent on the site of exposure to the antigen. Of the released inflammatory mediators, die most significant is histamine, which causes smooth muscle contraction and vascular permeability, and this in turn produces bronchoconstriction and edema. In addition, heparin, proteolytic enzymes, and neutrophil and eosinophil chemotactic factors are liberated. Mast cells also initiate formation of inflammatory mediators such as prostaglandins and leukotrienes (including slow-reacting substance of anaphylaxis). These contribute to reactions that develop several hours after exposure. Therefore, hypotension and even cardiovascular or respiratory arrest may occur.

Sequence of events in Type I Hypersensitivity reaction (Figs 3.1A and B):

- Allergen is inhaled/eaten/injected
- Allergen stimulates T_H2 production
- T_H2 cell secretes cytokines:
  - IL-4 stimulates B cells to make IgE
  - IL-5 recruits eosinophils
  - IL-13 stimulates mucous secretion
- Mast cell binds IgE
- Allergen bridges IgE on mast cell
- Mast cell degranulates.

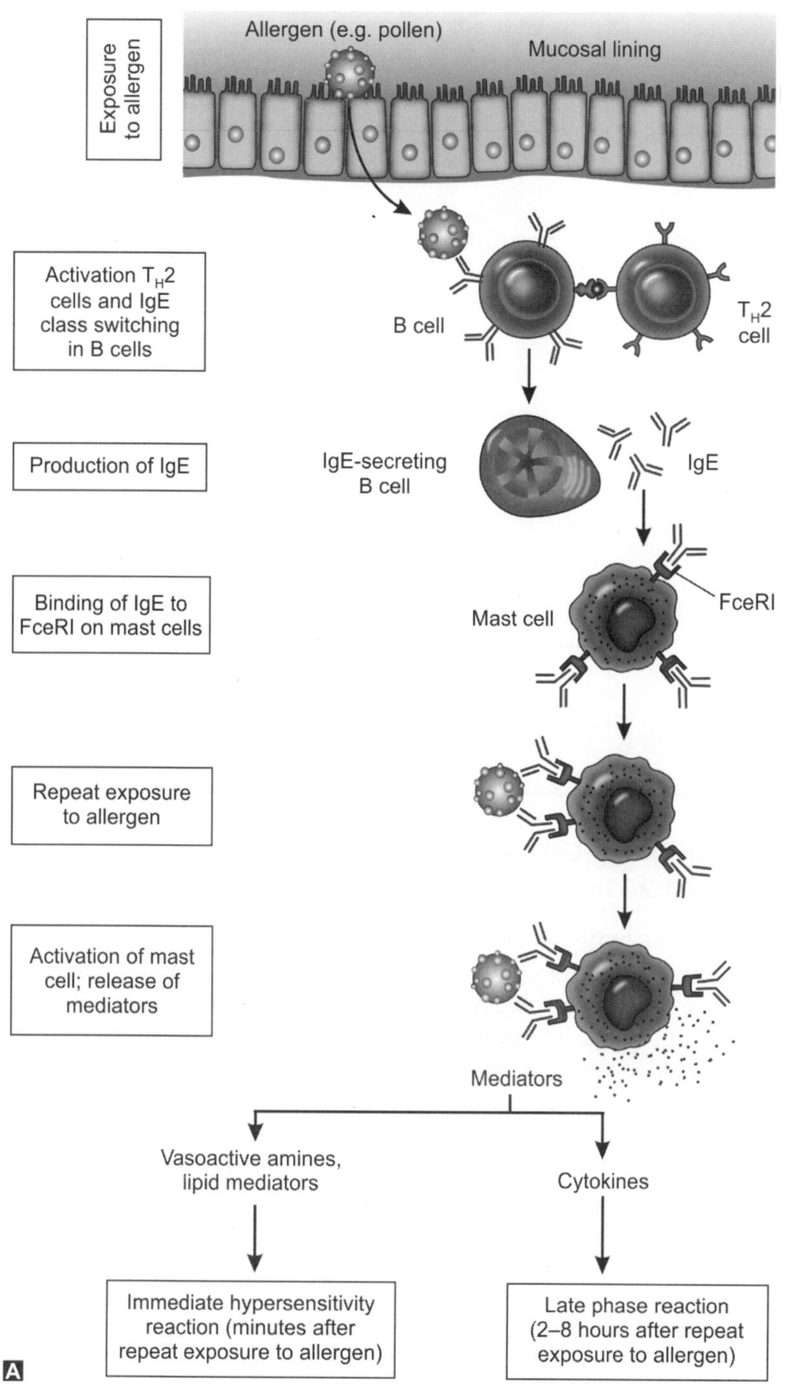

Exposure to allergen
Allergen (e.g. pollen)
Mucosal lining
Activation T_H2 cells and IgE class switching in B cells
B cell
T_H2 cell
Production of IgE
IgE-secreting B cell
IgE
Binding of IgE to FceRI on mast cells
Mast cell
FceRI
Repeat exposure to allergen
Activation of mast cell; release of mediators
Mediators
Vasoactive amines, lipid mediators
Cytokines
Immediate hypersensitivity reaction (minutes after repeat exposure to allergen)
Late phase reaction (2–8 hours after repeat exposure to allergen)
A

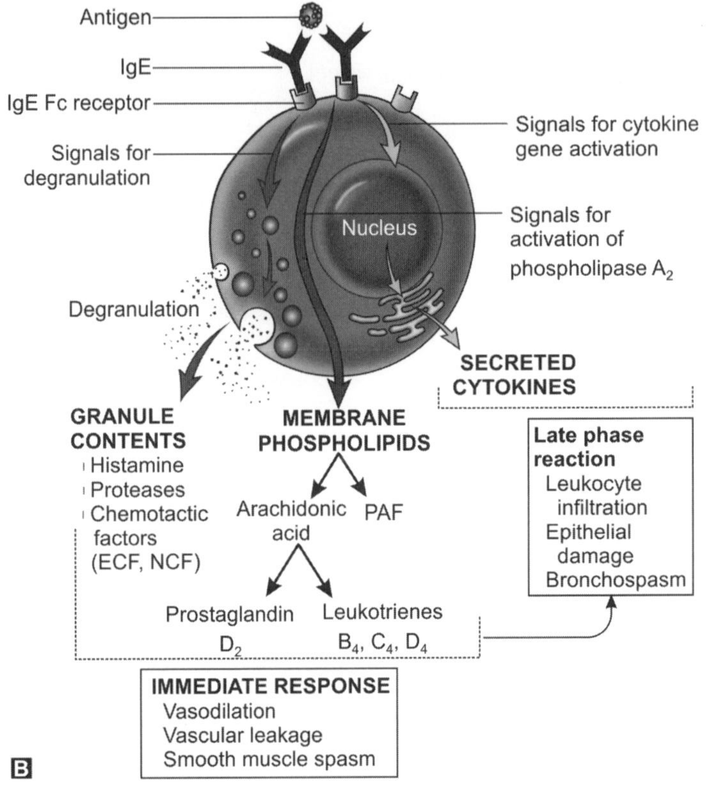

Figs 3.1A and B: Sequence of events in type I hypersensitivity reaction

Type II. Antibody-Cell Surface Reaction or Cytotoxic Hypersensitivity (Figs 3.2A to C)

In this type of hypersensitivity, cells are killed by the direct action of antibody against antigen on cell surfaces or in extracellular matrix, such as basement membrane. The suprabasilar split and acantholytic degenerating) cells in pemphigus and the infrabasilar split of a partially lysed basement membrane in pemphigoids are examples of this (Table 3.1). The antibody may also activate complements which leads to destruction of target cells by direct lysis (as of red blood cells in transfusion reactions) or indirectly by opsonization, as seen in some drug reactions. Other reactions are independent of complement, and the antibody that binds to the target cells may produce changes other than cell death within the cells.

This can be seen in autoimmune mediated hyperthyroidism (Graves' disease), where autoantibodies bind to thyroid stimulating hormone (TSH) receptor sites within the gland. The autoantibodies then simulate the effect of TSH itself the thyroid and cause an excess secretion of thyroid hormone.

Table 3.1: The diseases involved in type II hypersensitivity reaction

Disease	*Antigen*	*Symptoms*
Autoimmune hemolytic anemia	RBC antigens, drugs	Hemolysis
Pemphigus vulgaris	Proteins between epithelial cells	Bullae
Goodpasture syndrome	Proteins in glomeruli and alveoli	Nephritis, lung hemorrhage
Myasthenia gravis	Acetylcholine receptor	Muscle weakness
Graves disease	TSH receptor	Hyperthyroidism

Sequence of events in Type II Hypersensitivity reaction:

- Antibodies bind to cell-surface antigens
- One of three things happens:
  - Opsonization and phagocytosis
  - Inflammation
  - Cellular dysfunction.

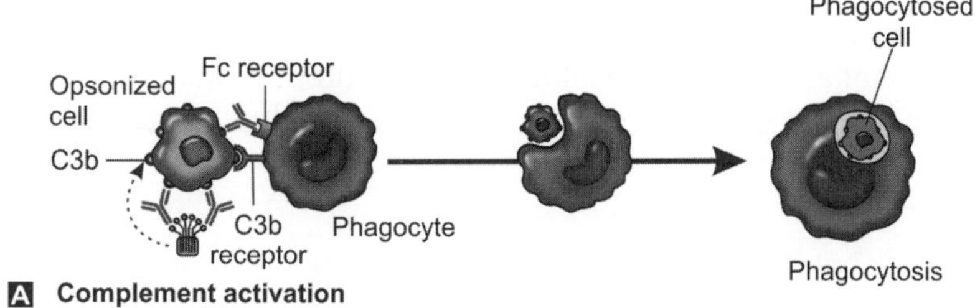

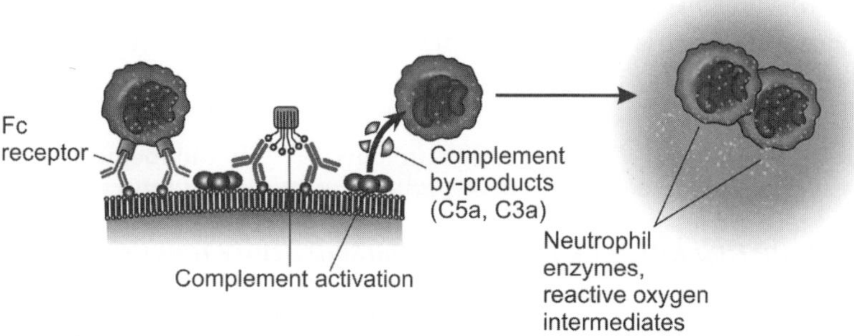

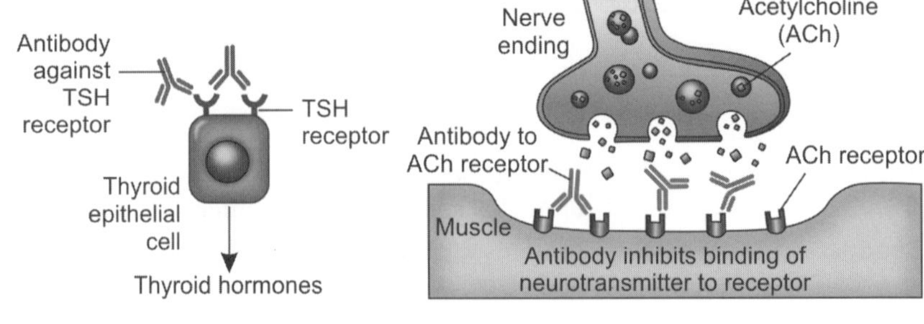

Figs 3.2A to C: Sequence of events in type II hypersensitivity reaction: (A) Opsonization and phagocytosis, (B) Complement and Fc receptor-mediated inflammation, (C) Antibody-mediated cellular dysfunction

Type III. Immune Complex Disease (Figs 3.3A to C)

In this type of reaction, tissue damage results from antigen-antibody complexes. Antibodies are formed against circulating or tissue-derived antigen. The resultant antigen-antibody complexes may be deposited in tissue, where they inflict damage by activating complement with a resultant influx of neutrophils and macrophages, which in turn release proteases and oxygen radicals. Deposits tend to occur in areas of high pressure and filtration, such as the kidney, and in diseases in which there is abundant antigen, such as infection and autoimmune disease. These include leprosy, bacterial endocarditis, systemic lupus erythematosus, rheumatoid arthritis, dermatomyositis and various forms of vasculitis (Table 3.2).

Table 3.2: The diseases involved in Type III hypersensitivity reaction

Disease	*Antigen*	*Symptoms*
Systemic lupus erythematosus	Nuclear antigens	Nephritis, skin lesions, arthritis...
Poststreptococcal glomerulonephritis	Streptococcal antigen	Nephritis
Polyarteritis nodosa	Hepatitis B antigen	Systemic vasculitis
Serum sickness	Foreign proteins	Arthritis, vasculitis, nephritis
Arthus reaction	Foreign proteins	Cutaneous vasculitis

There are two kinds of Type III Hypersensitivity reaction:

- Systemic immune complex disease
  - Complexes formed in circulation
  - Deposited in several organs
  - Example: Serum sickness.

- Local immune complex disease
  - Complexes formed at site of antigen injection
  - Precipitated at injection site
  - Example: Arthus reaction.

TYPE III. HYPERSENSITIVITY REACTION

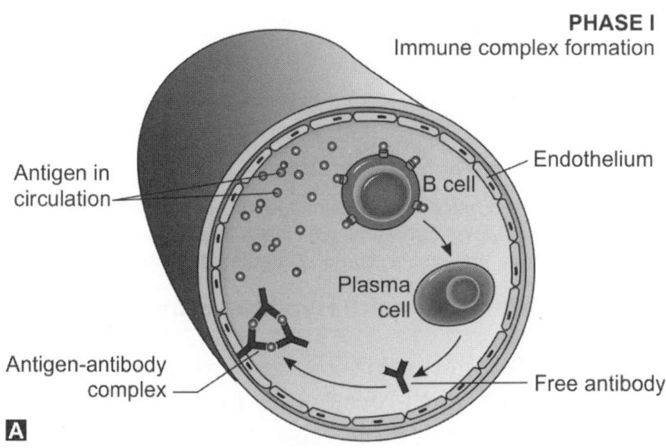

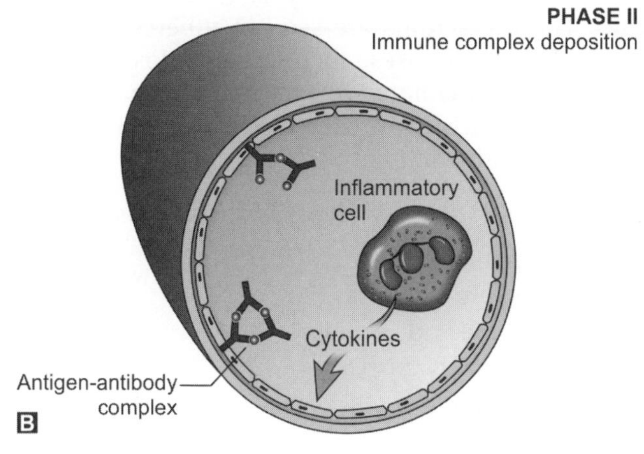

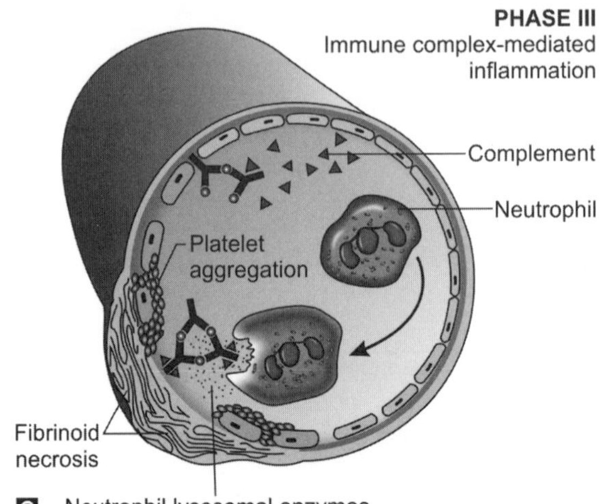

Figs 3.3A to C: Sequence of events in type III hypersensitivity reaction—(A) Phase I: Immune complex formation, (B) Phase II: Immune complex deposition, (C) Phase III: Immune complex-mediated inflammation

Type IV. Cell-Mediated (Delayed) Hypersensitivity (Figs 3.4A and B)

Antigen-reactive cells, not antibody, are involved in cell-mediated hypersensitivities. Antigen is processed by macrophages or Langerhans cells and presented to antigen-specific T lymphocytes. The activted cells release lymphokines, which recruit and activate lymphocytes, macrophages, and fibroblasts. Injury is induced by T cells and/or macrophages. These reactions are seen in tuberculin hypersensitivity and in granulomatous diseases, such as sarcoidosis and tuberculosis. Other examples of cell-mediated hypersensitivity include lichen planus and contact hypersensitivity, in which the Langerhans cells within the epithelium play a significant role.

There are two kinds of Type IV Hypersensitivity reaction (Fig. 3.5):

- Delayed-type hypersensitivity (DTH)
  - CD4+ T cells secrete cytokines
  - Macrophages come and kill cells
- Direct cell cytotoxicity
  - CD8+ T cells kill targeted cells

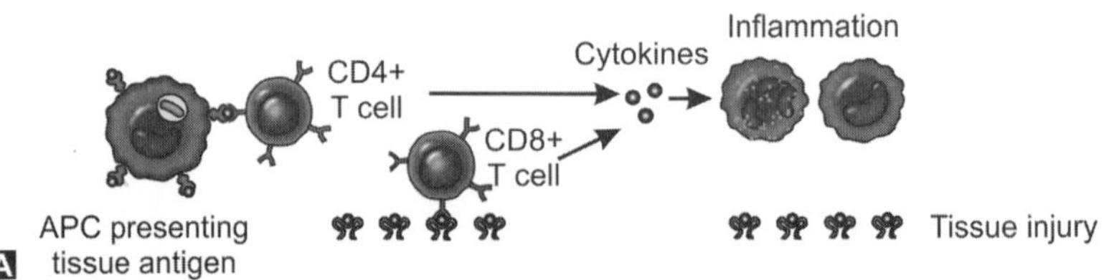

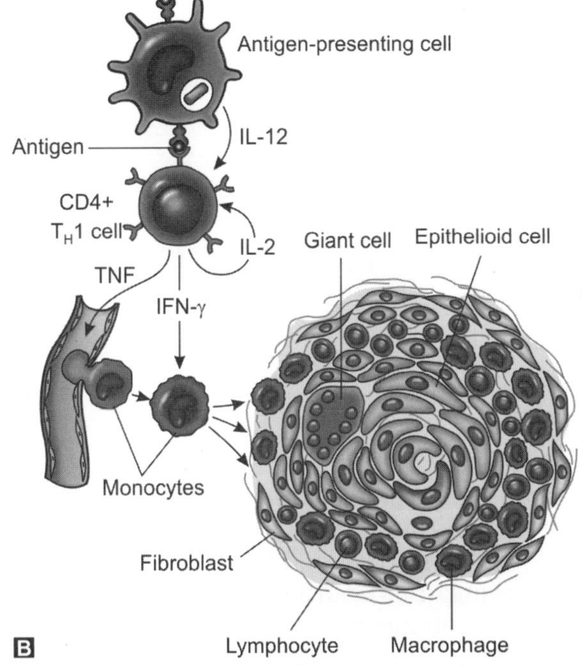

Figs 3.4A and B: Delayed-type hypersensitivity

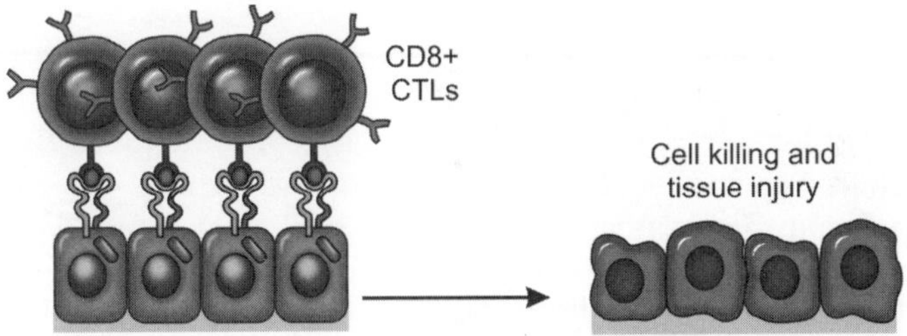

Fig. 3.5: T-cell-mediated cytotoxicity

CHAPTER 4

Oral Lichen Planus

INTRODUCTION[1]

Oral lichen planus (OLP) is a chronic inflammatory disorder affecting stratified squamous epithelia. The disease is relatively common, affecting approximately 1–2% of the population, an incidence equal to well-known diseases such as psoriasis and Barrett's esophagus.

Whereas in the majority of instances, cutaneous lesions of lichen planus (LP) are self-limiting and cause itching, oral lesions in OLP are chronic, rarely undergo spontaneous remission, are potentially premalignant and are often a source of morbidity. Furthermore, oral lesions, unlike cutaneous lesions, are difficult to palliate (Figs 4.1 and 4.2).

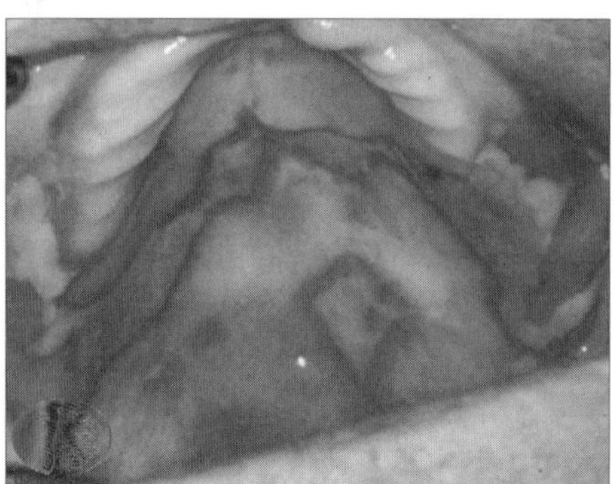

Fig. 4.1: OLP due to drug reaction

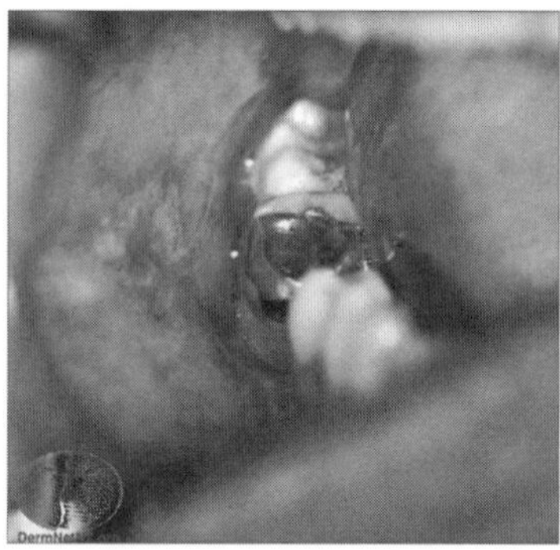

Fig. 4.2: OLP reaction to amalgam

ETIOLOGY AND PATHOGENESIS[3]

The cause of LP is not known but immunologic mechanisms triggered by poorly defined antigenic stimulations plays a pivotal role in the pathogenesis of the disease. Cell-mediated immune response is believed to play the major role in the pathology of the disease. Presence of activated antigen presenting cells (Langerhans cells, dendritic macrophages) in the lesional skin could be demonstrated in the early stage of the disease.

$CD4^+$ cells initiates immune response in which activated keratinocytes also take part. $CD8^+$ T lymphocytes mediate the damage to the epidermis and leads to the characteristic lichenoid tissue reaction.

There is evidence of the role of HLA-associated genetic susceptibility in the causation of the disease.

There are cases of lichen planus-type rashes (known as lichenoid reactions) occurring as allergic reactions to medications for high blood pressure, heart disease and arthritis. These lichenoid reactions are referred to as *lichenoid mucositis* (*of the mucosa*) or *dermatitis* (*of the skin*).

Contact allergens in dental restorative materials or toothpastes (contact hypersensitivity reactions).

Mechanical trauma (*Koebner phenomenon*) (Fig. 4.3).

Lichen planus has been reported as a complication of chronic *hepatitis C virus* infection and can be a sign of *chronic graft-versus-host disease* of the skin (Fig. 4.4).

It has been suggested that true lichen planus may respond to stress, where lesions may present on the mucosa or skin during times of stress in those with the disease.

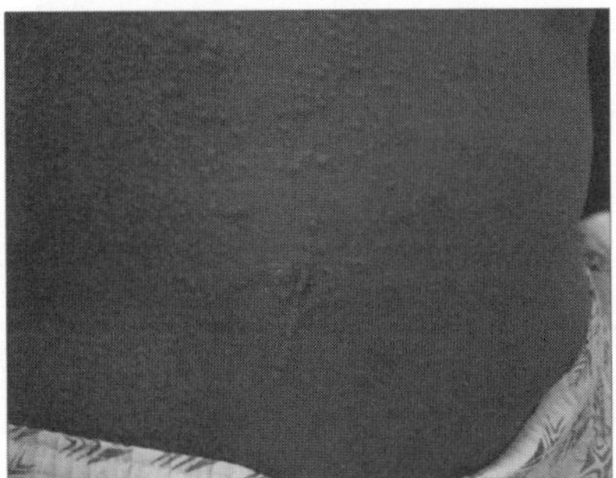

Fig. 4.3: Koebner phenomenon

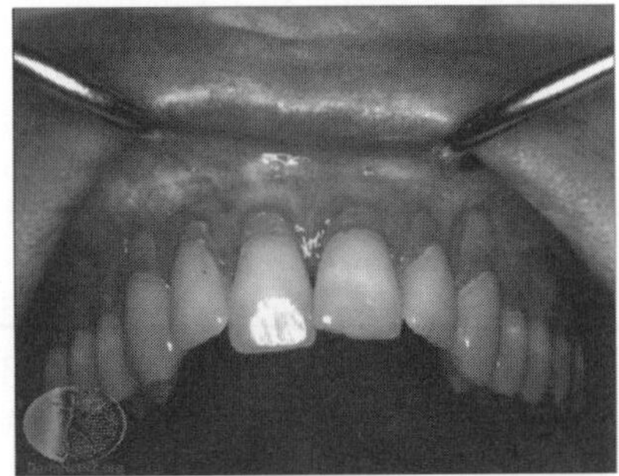

Fig. 4.4: Graft-verses-host disease

CLINICAL FEATURES[1]

OLP develops most commonly in the 5th to 6th decades of life, and in women more than twice as often as in men, patients of all ages may develop the disorder.

Extraoral Manifestations

Patients with OLP frequently have concomitant disease in one or more extraoral sites. Therefore, a thorough evaluation and multidisciplinary approach is required to uncover potential sites of extraoral involvement.

Approximately 15% of patients with OLP develop cutaneous lesions. The classic appearance of skin lesions consists of erythematous to violaceous papules that are flat-topped and occasionally polygonal in form (Fig. 4.5). A network of fine lines (Wickham striae) often overlies many of the papules. Cutaneous LP may also appear in several atypical forms that are not easily recognizable.

Typically, cutaneous lesions develop within several months after the appearance of the oral lesions, and the severity of the oral lesions does not seem to correlate with the extent of cutaneous involvement.

Undoubtedly, the most frequent extraoral site of involvement in female patients with OLP is the genital mucosa with lesions developing in 20% of women with OLP. The association of LP of the vulva, vagina and gingiva is recognized as the vulvovaginal-gingival syndrome. When LP affects the genital mucosa, the erosive form of the disease is the predominant type (Fig. 4.6) although asymptomatic reticular lesions can be identified in a quarter of all patients. Various symptoms including burning, pain, vaginal discharge, and dyspareunia are frequent and are noted in patients with erythematous and erosive disease. Not uncommonly, patients with mild oral involvement display severe erosive vulvovaginal disease, and patients afflicted with severe oral involvement develop only mild asymptomatic genital disease. Reports of malignant transformation of genital lichen planus in women underscore the need for an early diagnosis and the institution of prompt treatment for these patients.

The penogingival syndrome represents the male equivalent of the vulvovaginal-gingival syndrome of LP. Although the concomitant involvement of oral and genital LP is much less common in males than females, recognition and treatment of the disease are important as malignant transformation of penile LP has been reported.

Lichen planopilaris represents LP involvement of the scalp and hair follicles causing a scarring alopecia. Lichen planus may also involve the nails producing thinning and ridging of the nail plate and splitting of the distal free edge of the nail. Healing with a scar produces a pterygium, an uncommon but characteristic LP nail manifestation. Lichen planus of the nails and scalp are uncommon in patients with OLP.

The clinical features of esophageal LP have been well documented, and the disease appears to develop most commonly in patients with OLP.

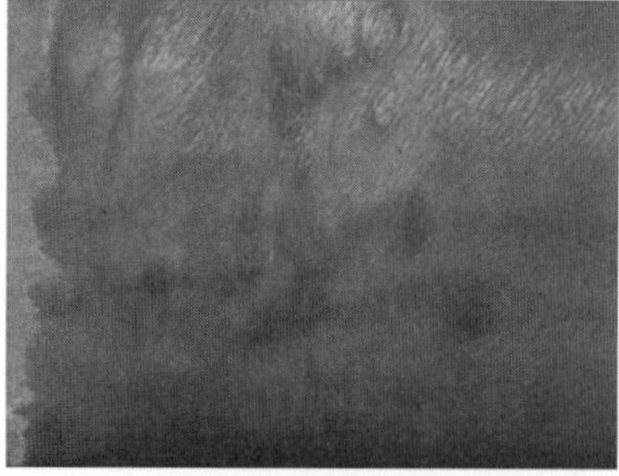

Fig. 4.5: Cutaneous LP: Violaceous papules that are flat-topped and polygonal in form covered with a network of fine lines (Wickham striae)

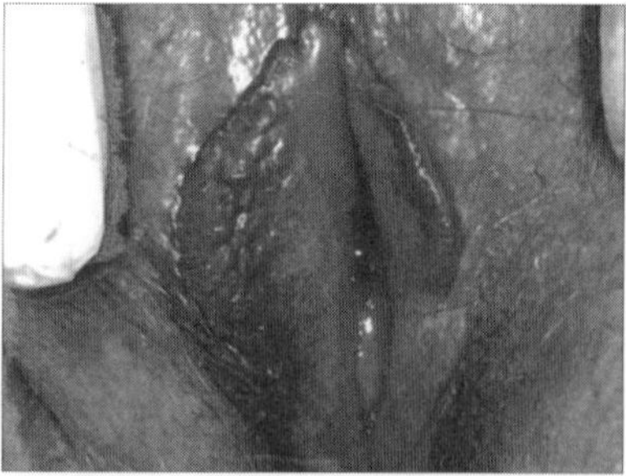

Fig. 4.6: Vulvovaginal LP: The characteristic lesion is a tender, painful, erythematous atrophic or eroded introitus of the vulvovaginal area

The overwhelming majority of patients with esophageal LP are diagnosed as a result of painful symptoms, with dysphagia being the predominant complaint. Although malignant transformation has not been reported, untreated esophageal LP may result in chronic pain and strictures. Patients with OLP may also develop the disease in one or more sites including the ocular, bladder, nasal, laryngeal, otic, gastric, and anal structures although these sites of involvement are uncommon.

ORAL MANIFESTATIONS[1]

Oral lichen planus lesions usually have recognizable and distinctive clinical features and a characteristic distribution. OLP may manifest in one of three clinical forms: Reticular, erythematous (atrophic) and erosive (ulcerated, bullous). Whereas reticular lesions occur as isolated lesions and are often the only clinical manifestation of the disease, erythematous lesions are accompanied by reticular lesions, and erosive lesions are accompanied by reticular and erythematous lesions in almost all cases. This feature helps clinically differentiate OLP from other vesiculo-erosive diseases such as pemphigus and pemphigoid, which are characterized by isolated areas of erythema and/or erosions.

The **reticular lesions**, the most recognized form of OLP, encompass white lesions, which appear as a network of connecting and overlapping lines (Wickham striae), papules or plaques (Fig. 4.7). Although some patients may display an impressive array of diffuse and widespread reticulated lesions, they rarely complain of symptoms and often, are unaware of their presence.

Erythematous (Fig. 4.8) **and erosive** (Fig. 4.9) OLP lesions result in varying degrees of discomfort. The number of ulcerations is variable as are their size and location; rarely, bulla that ruptures easily may be observed in the erosive form of OLP. The erosive lesions hardly ever remit spontaneously and may lead to confusion with other autoimmune mucosal, vesiculoerosive diseases, which share similar clinical features.

The posterior buccal mucosa is the most frequent site of involvement followed by the tongue, gingiva, labial mucosa, and vermilion of

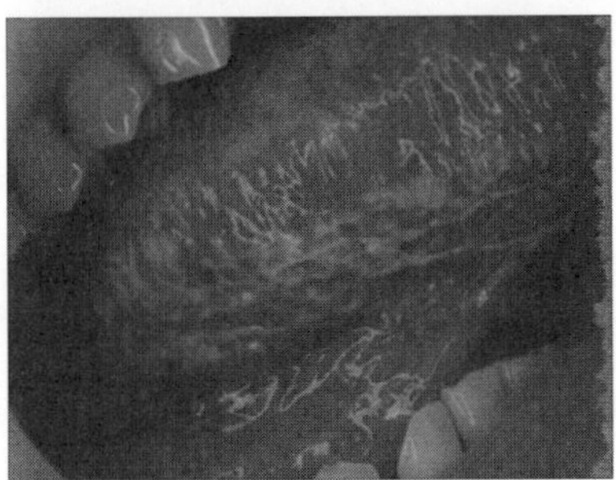

Fig. 4.7: Reticular lesions may be papular, plaque-like, and lacy and are the most recognized form of OLP

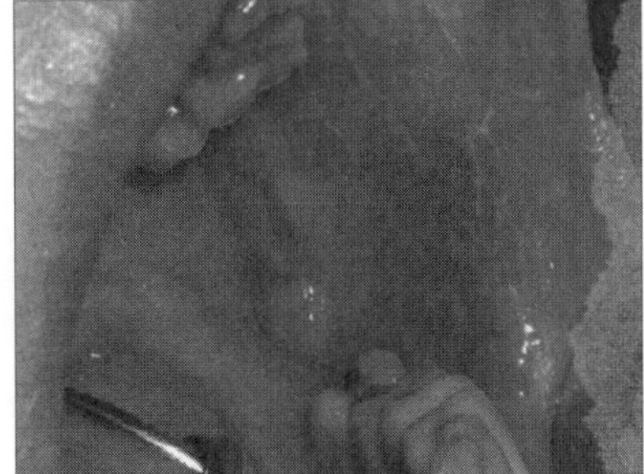

Fig. 4.8: Erythematous OLP lesions, when present, are almost always accompanied by reticulated lesions

the lower lip. Lesions on the palate, floor of the mouth, and upper lip are uncommonly noted.

Approximately 10% of patients with OLP have the disease confined to the gingiva. Gingival LP presenting as small, raised white, lacy papules or plaques, may resemble keratotic diseases such as leukoplakia. Erythematous lesions affecting the gingiva result in desquamative gingivitis (Fig. 4.10), the most common type of gingival LP. Erosive lesions resembling those observed in other vesiculoerosive diseases including pemphigoid, pemphigus, linear IgA disease, and foreign body gingivitis also produce desquamative gingivitis not easily identified as lichen planus unless there are coexistent reticular lesions on the gingiva or elsewhere in the oral cavity.

Lichen planus isolated to a single oral site other than the gingiva is uncommon. Patients with isolated lip lesions and tongue lesions have been described although many patients who present with isolated lesions eventually develop more widespread disease.

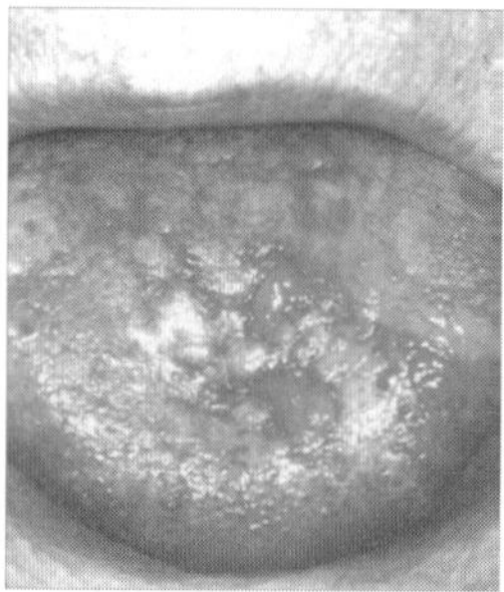

Fig. 4.9: The most severe and painful lesions of OLP develop in the erosive form of the disease

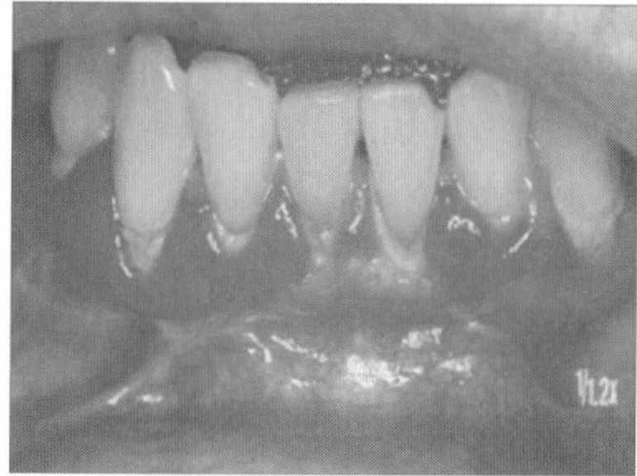

Fig. 4.10: OLP confined to the gingiva, typically with atrophic and erosive lesions resulting in desquamative gingivitis

CLASSIFICATION

Andreason in 1968 divided OLP into 6 clinical forms:
Atrophic (erythematous)
Reticular
Erosive (ulcerated)
Bullous
Papular and Plaque-like.

The bullous form: It presents as fluid-filled vesicles which project from the surface.

The hypertrophic form: It may also appear on the oral mucosa, generally appearing as a well-circumscribed, elevated white lesion resembling leukoplakia (Fig. 4.11).

Atrophic (erythematous): It appears clinically as smooth, red, poorly defined areas; often but not always with the peripheral striae evident. It usually occurs on the gingiva (Fig. 4.12).

Papular and Plaque-like: It confluents white patches similar to oral keratosis; usually seen in smokers (Fig. 4.13).

Histologic Features:[2] Basal epidermal keratinocyte damage and lichenoid-interface lymphocytic reaction are the two major pathological findings. There are presence of hyperkeratosis, increased granular layer, irregular acanthosis, liquefactive degeneration of the basal cell layer and band-like lymphocytic infiltrate in the upper dermis. In mucosal lichen planus, plasma cells are more prominent. Degenerated keratinocytes (colloid, Civatte bodies) are present at the dermal-epidermal junction (Fig. 4.14, Table 4.1).

Direct immunofluorescence shows heavy deposits of fibrin at the dermo-epidermal junction. Deposits of IgM and less frequently IgG, IgA and C3 are also found in the colloid bodies (Fig. 4.15).

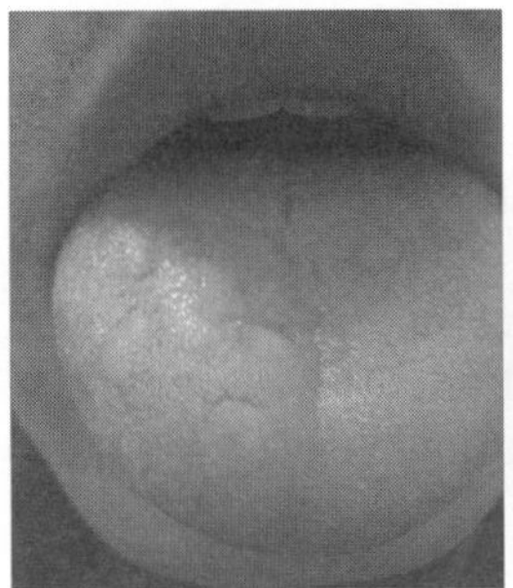

Fig. 4.11: Hypertropic OLP

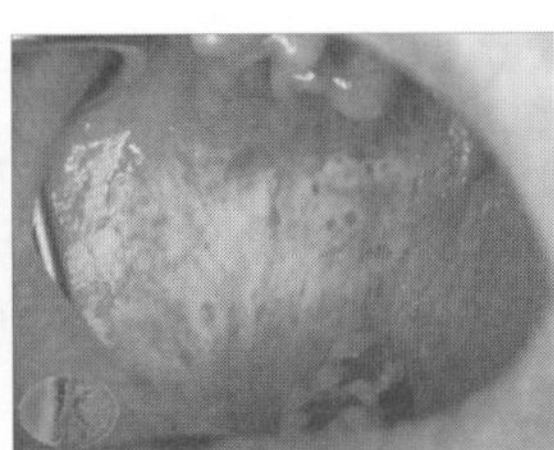

Fig. 4.12: Atrophic OLP

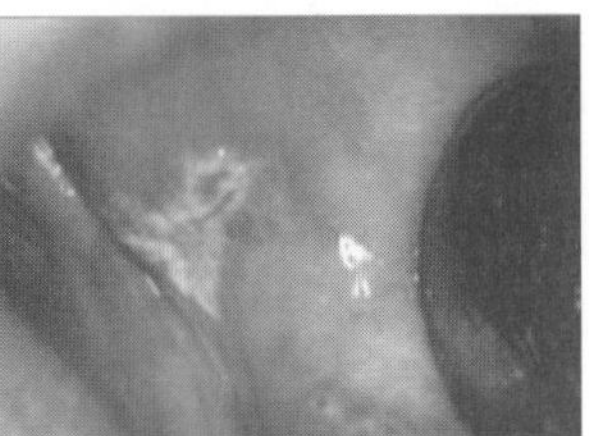

Fig. 4.13: Plaque-like OLP

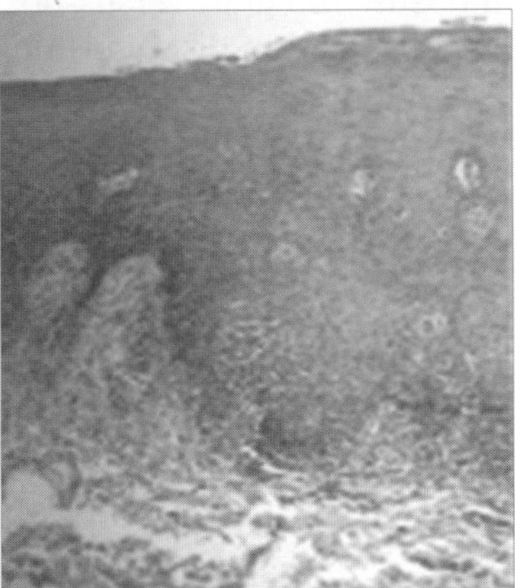

Fig. 4.14: Hyperkeratosis, saw toothed rete ridges, and a band-like infiltrate of lymphocytes subjacent to the epithelium

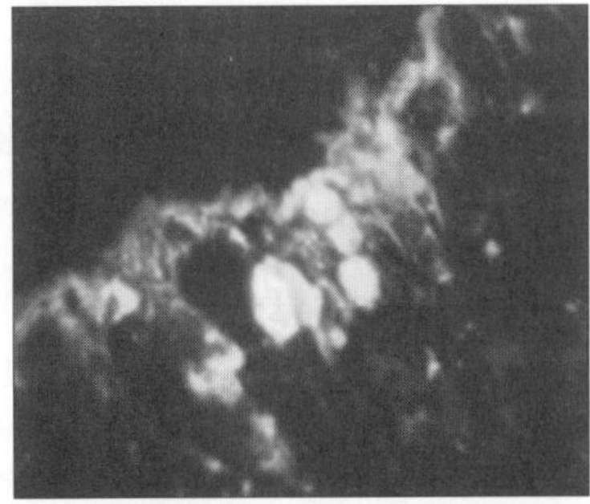

Fig. 4.15: Direct immunofluorescence shows heavy deposits of fibrin at the dermoepidermal junction

Table 4.1: Histopathologic and immunofluorescent features OLP

Table 4.1: Histopathologic and immunofluorescent features OLP
Histology (Eisenberg, 2000)
Essential features
Superficial band-like infiltrate of T lymphocytes
Basal cell liquefaction degeneration
Normal epithelial maturation pattern
Additional features
Jagged, spindly rete ridges
Civatte bodies
Separation of epithelium from lamina propria
Immunofluorescence of perilesional mucosa (Helander and Rogers, 1994)
Fibrin and shaggy fibrinogen in a linear pattern at the basement membrane zone
Cytoids in the absence of deposition of fibrinogen.

Lichen planus may also affect the genital mucosa—vulvovaginal-gingival lichen planus. It can resemble other skin conditions such as atopic dermatitis and psoriasis.

Rarely, lichen planus shows esophageal involvement, where it can present with erosive esophagitis and stricturing. It has also been hypothesized that it is a precursor to squamous cell carcinoma of the esophagus.

DIFFERENTIAL DIAGNOSIS[2]

The clinical differential diagnosis include lichenoid drug reactions, lichenoid reactions associated with contact hypersensitivity to restorative materials, leukoplakia, lupus erythematosus, and graft-versus-host disease (GVHD). Direct immunofluorescence can aid in distinguishing OLP from other lesions specially from vesiculobullous lesions such as pemphigus vulgaris, benign mucous membrane pemphigoid, and linear IgA bullous dermatosis.

MANAGEMENT[2] (FLOWCHART 4.1)

In general, nonerosive oral lichen planus is asymptomatic and treatment is often unnecessary. However, patients with erosive type oral lichen planus often present with significant management problems. At present, none of the available treatment is specific or universally effective. An algorithm for the management of oral lichen planus is shown. All patients should optimize their oral hygiene. Oral candidiasis should be excluded or treated accordingly. In symptomatic patients with apparent contact dental factor, patch test with replacement of the amalgam or gold restorative material is suggested in those who are sensitized to these metals. In those with no apparent contact factor, topical or intralesional steroid is usually the first line treatment. A short course of systemic steroid may be necessary for more rapid control. In steroid-dependent patients, azathioprine or topical cyclosporine can be added as an adjunctive therapy. In refractory cases, alternative therapies such as topical or systemic retinoids, antimalarial, dapsone, oral PUVA, thalidomide or topical tacrolimus may be considered. Surgical treatments such as laser, cryotherapy and excision may exacerbate the conditions due to the Koebner phenomenon.

Note: *Oral lichen planus presenting as atrophic, erosive or bullous clinical types are usually symptomatic and refractory to treatments. In patients with oral lichenoid lesions, drug eruption due to oral medications or dental contact factor should be eliminated.*

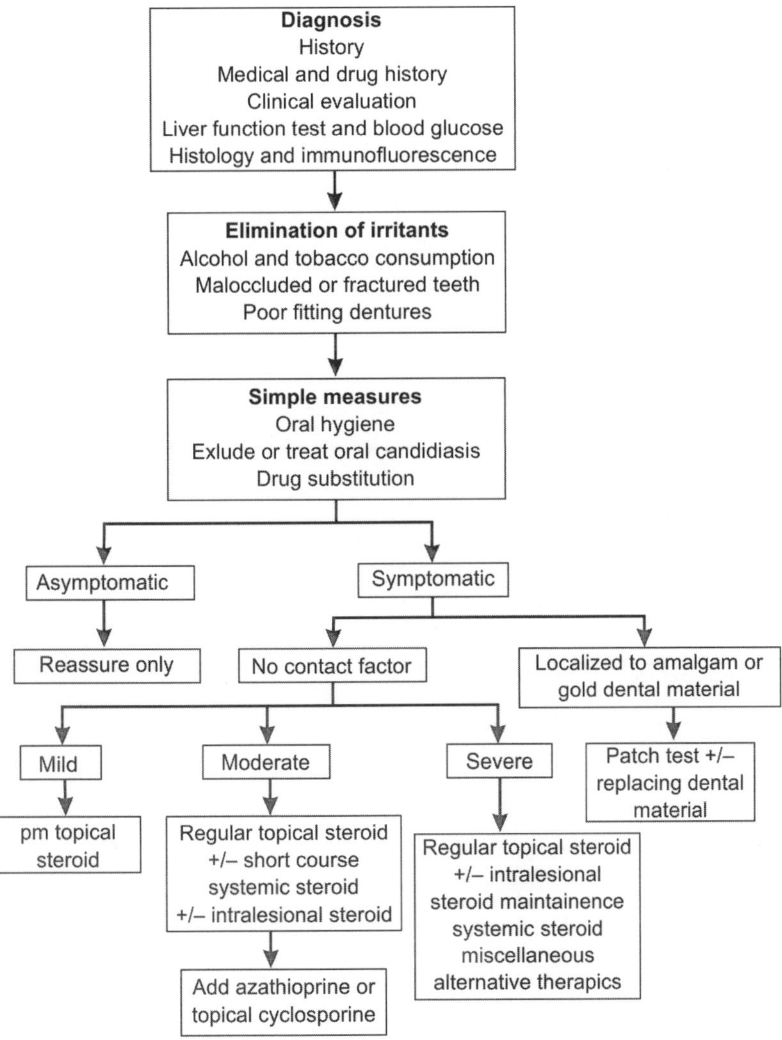

Flowchart 4.1: Management of lichen planus

REFERENCES

1. Eisen D, Carrozzo M, Bagan Sebastian JV, Thongprasom K. Oral lichen planus: Clinical features and management. Mucosal Diseases Series, Oral Diseases 2005;11(5):338–49.
2. Cheng SY. Oral lichen planus, Hong Kong Dermatology & Venereology Bulletin. 13 March, 2002.

CHAPTER

5

Systemic Sclerosis

(**Synonyms**: Scleroderma, progressive systemic sclerosis)

INTRODUCTION[1]

Systemic sclerosis (SSc) is characterized by progressive fibrosis of skin and multiple organs. The term 'scleroderma' literally means 'hard skin' (sclera—hard; derma—skin). Though the term scleroderma is indelibly etched in the literature through the common usage, the disease is currently called as "systemic sclerosis". Since hidebound skin is the hallmark of the disease, it is also called as "hidebound disease".

PATHOGENESIS[4]

Pathological changes in SSc encompass a spectrum reflecting variable stages of development and progression of 3 major processes in the affected tissues:

1. Severe tissue fibrosis with exaggerated deposition of collagen and other connective tissue components in the extracellular matrix.
2. Chronic inflammation, occurring predominantly in the early stages of disease and characterized by infiltration with mononuclear cells, mostly of the macrophage and T-cell lineages.
3. Microvascular disease, characterized by intimal proliferation, concentric subendothelial deposition of collagen and mucinous material, and narrowing and thrombosis of the vessel lumen.

The underlying physiologic basis for the diffuse vasculopathy in SSc is unknown. Initial events are thought to involve endothelial cell injury, with subsequent loss of normal vasodilatory mediators including prostacyclin and nitric oxide. As a result, abnormal responses to vasoconstrictive mediators, including catecholamines, may occur. Endothelial injury also leads to increased release of endothelin 1 (ET-1), which is a 21-amino acid peptide released by endothelial cells that has a potent vasoconstrictive effect. It binds to 2 cognate receptors, ET-A and ET-B, which are variably expressed on endothelial cells, smooth muscle cells, fibroblasts and other cells throughout the body. ET-1 is found in increased levels in the serum of patients with SSc, suggesting that it plays a role in the pathogenesis of SSc vascular disease. Like Raynaud's phenomenon, pulmonary hypertension in these patients is characterized by both functional and structural abnormalities, and the structural lesion in pulmonary hypertension resembles the vascular lesion in SSc associated Raynaud's (Flowchart 5.1).

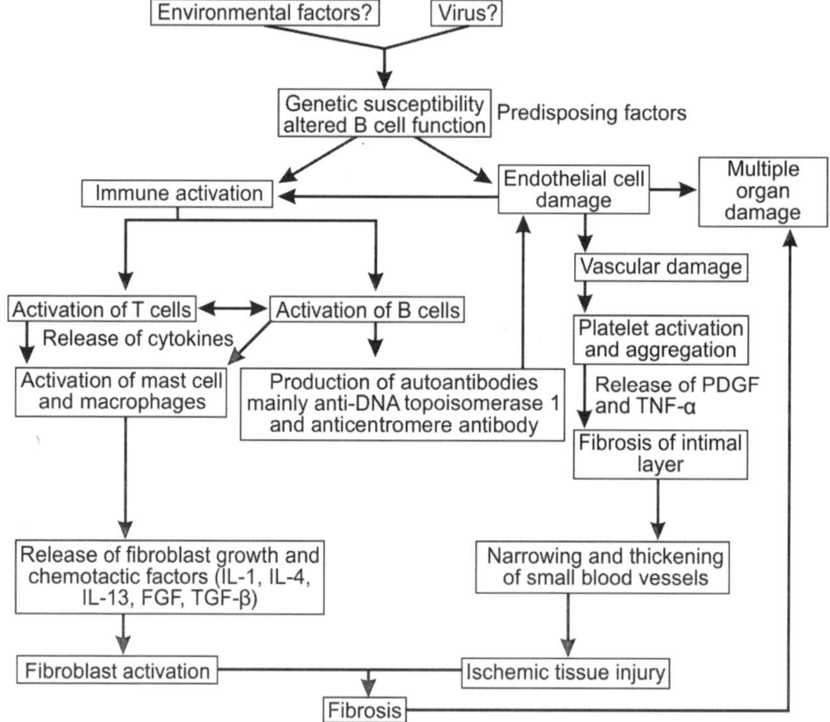

Flowchart 5.1: Pathogenesis of systemic sclerosis

CLINICAL FEATURES

SSc is an autoimmune disease, characterized by widespread fibrosis of subcutaneous connective tissue, which can cause serious complications, with the involvement of other systems. The greatest incidence of the disease occurs between the ages of 30 years and 50 years, and women are affected about 3 times as often as men.[2]

CLASSIFICATION

According to its pace, the disease is classified into 2 major subsets (Flowchart 5.2):[2]

(1) Limited cutaneous SSc (the old CREST syndrome)
(2) Diffuse cutaneous SSc.

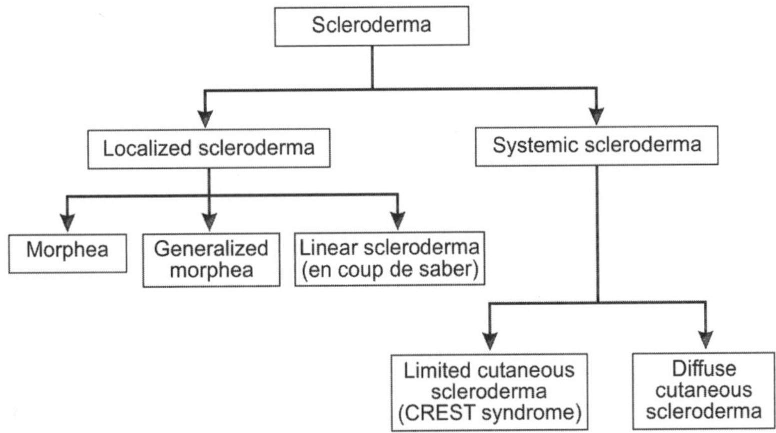

Flowchart 5.2: Classification of systemic sclerosis

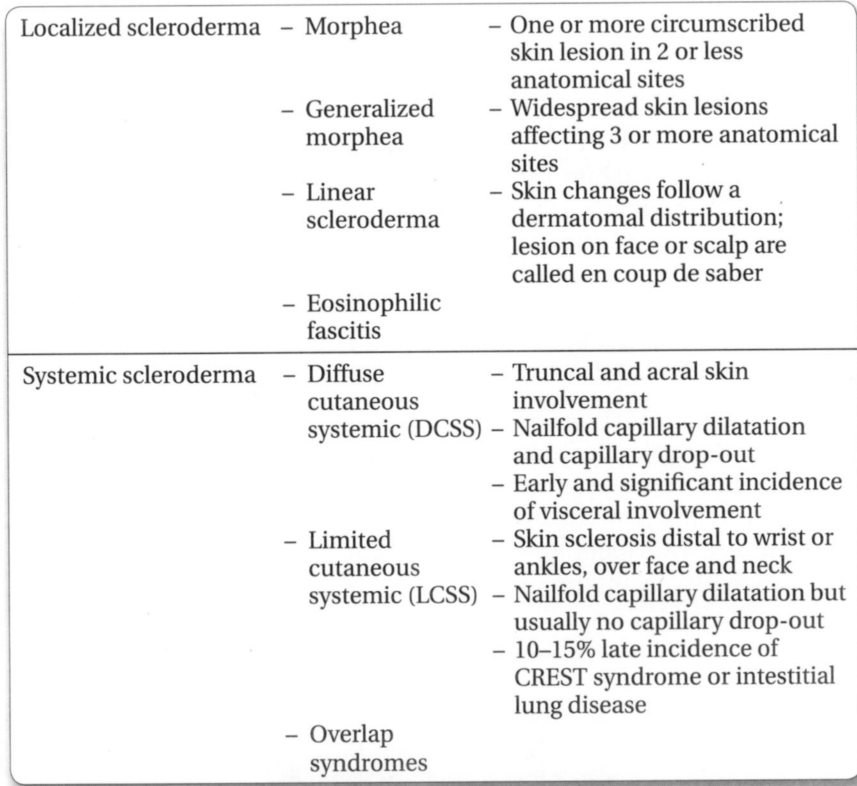

Localized scleroderma	– Morphea	– One or more circumscribed skin lesion in 2 or less anatomical sites
	– Generalized morphea	– Widespread skin lesions affecting 3 or more anatomical sites
	– Linear scleroderma	– Skin changes follow a dermatomal distribution; lesion on face or scalp are called en coup de saber
	– Eosinophilic fascitis	
Systemic scleroderma	– Diffuse cutaneous systemic (DCSS)	– Truncal and acral skin involvement – Nailfold capillary dilatation and capillary drop-out – Early and significant incidence of visceral involvement
	– Limited cutaneous systemic (LCSS)	– Skin sclerosis distal to wrist or ankles, over face and neck – Nailfold capillary dilatation but usually no capillary drop-out – 10–15% late incidence of CREST syndrome or intestitial lung disease
	– Overlap syndromes	

Limited SSc patients usually have a long history of Raynaud's phenomenon prior to other symptoms, such as skin thickening limited to hands, digital ulcers, esophageal dysmotility, small intestine hypomotility and pulmonary hypertension.

Diffuse SSc patients have a rather acute onset with symptoms such as arthritis, carpal tunnel syndrome, marked swelling of hands and legs and widespread skin thickening progressing from the fingers to the trunk. Involvement of organs and systems other than the skin is extremely common and is often discovered either concomitantly with initial diagnosis of the cutaneous disorder, or on future evaluation. In addition to internal organ problems that include gastrointestinal and pulmonary fibrosis, severe life-threatening involvement of the heart and kidneys has also been reported in diffuse SSc patients.[2]

Bone resorption has been reported when SSc reaches a more advanced state and it has been reported on the terminal phalanges, the distal radius and the ulna, the cervical spine, the zygomatic arch, the ribs and the mandible. The exact cause of this finding is unknown; however, it is known that the majority of SSc patients have characteristic diffuse sclerotic atrophy of the skin, which progresses into a fibrotic form and becomes tightly bound to the subcutaneous structures. The tight, firm skin causes extrinsic pressure and the obliteration of vessels, consequently leading to ischemia and destruction of the underlying bone. This mechanism may also lead to bone resorption of the mandibular body, as it affects the other bones of the skeleton.[2]

Deposition of calcium salts (calcinosis) in the skin and subcutaneous tissue occurs in a variety of rheumatic diseases, including SSc. Calcinosis is generally classified into 4 subsets: Dystrophic, metastatic, idiopathic or calciphylaxis/iatrogenic, and its pathophysiology still remains unclear.

Focal and diffuse subcutaneous calcifications may develop in 20–30% of SSc patients with the CREST syndrome and are commonly seen on fingertips and over bony eminences.[2]

ORAL MANIFESTATIONS

The oral and perioral tissues are also commonly involved. Most common dental finding in SSc include the widening of the periodontal ligament (PDL) space in the absence of a significant periodontal infection (Fig. 5.1). Additionally, it has been shown that despite the widening of the PDL space, the involved teeth were often not mobile and their gingival attachments were usually intact.[2]

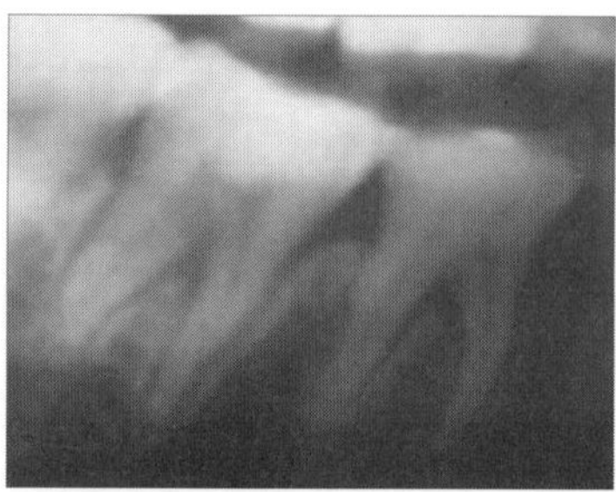

Fig. 5.1: Widening of the periodontal ligament space around the roots of the posterior teeth

Other findings include rigid lips, narrow oral aperture, loss of skin folds around the mouth (mask-like appearance), blanching of the oral mucosa due to fibrosis (Figs 5.2 and 5.3), and sclerosis of the tongue (Fig. 5.4), oral telangiectasia, and pseudoankylosis. Oral and perioral effects are mainly caused by skin and muscular atrophy seen in these patients. Xerostomia is also commonly seen in patients with systemic sclerosis and is either caused by glandular fibrosis or is found to be associated with Sjögren's syndrome. Resorption of the mandible in areas of masticatory muscle attachments (angle, condyle, coronoid, and digastric) has also been reported.[3]

HISTOLOGIC FEATURES[5]

Microscopic examination of tissue involved by systemic sclerosis shows diffuse deposition of dense collagen within and around the normal structures (Fig. 5.5). This abnormal collagen replaces and destroys the normal tissue, causing the loss of normal tissue function. The loss of dermal appendages, particularly the sweat glands, and atrophy of the epithelium with loss of retepegs and increased melanin pigmentation are seen.

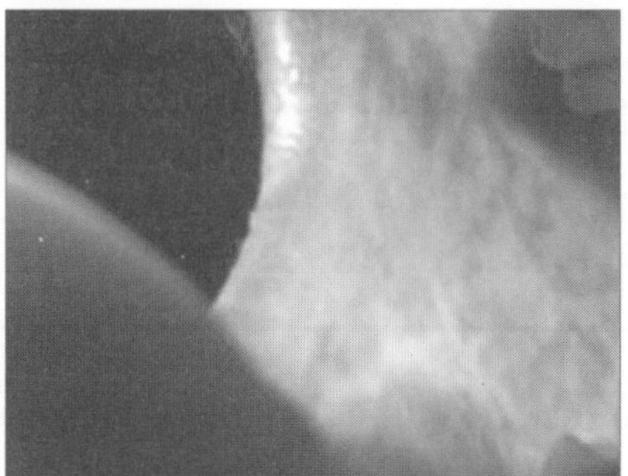

Fig. 5.2: Blanching of the oral mucosa due to fibrosis

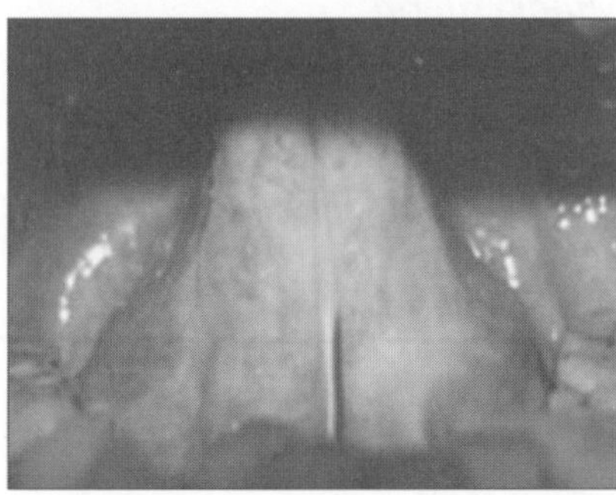

Fig. 5.3: Blanching of the ventral surface of the tongue with thickening of the lingual frenum

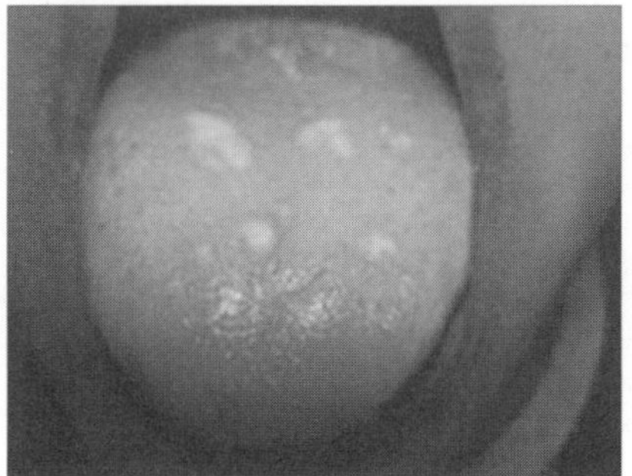

Fig. 5.4: Depapillation of the tongue due to fibrosis

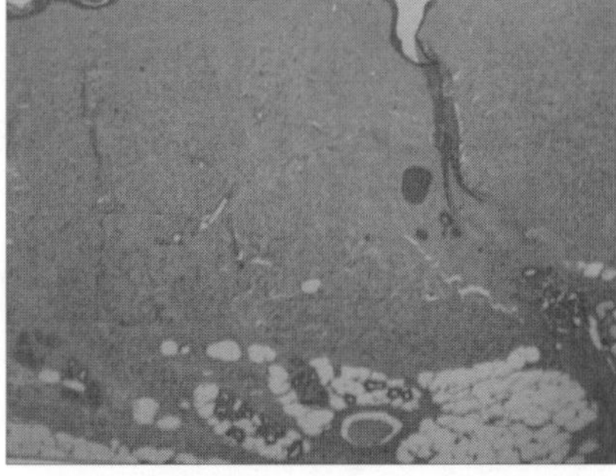

Fig. 5.5: Excessive deposition of collagen extending into the fat. The overlying epithelium and skin appendages are atrophic

DIAGNOSIS[5]

During early phases, it may be difficult to make a diagnosis of systemic sclerosis. Generally, the clinical signs of stiffened skin texture along with the development of Raynaud's phenomenon are suggestive of the diagnosis.

A skin biopsy may be supportive of the diagnoses if abundant collagen deposition is observed microscopically. Laboratory studies may be helpful to the diagnostic process if anticentromere antibodies or anti-Scl 70 (topoisomerase I) is detected. Anti-Scl 70 antibodies are seen more often with systemic sclerosis; anticentromere antibodies are usually associated with more limited forms of scleroderma or CREST syndrome. In addition, increasing levels of autoantibodies appear to correlate with disease severity.

American Rheumatism Association Diagnostic Criteria for Progressive Systemic Sclerosis

Major criteria
Proximal sclerosis (91% sensitivity and greater than 99% specificity).
Minor criteria
Sclerodactyly.
Digital pitting scars of finger tips or loss of substance of finger pad.
Pulmonary fibrosis-bibasilar.
Note: *One major or two minor criteria were found in 97% of patients with definite systemic sclerosis.*

TREATMENT[6]

There is no adequate treatment for progressive diffuse systemic sclerosis, although partial remissions have been reported following cortisone therapy. Circumscribed scleroderma has an excellent prognosis, since spontaneous.

REFERENCES

1. Ahathya RS, Deepalakshmi D, Emmadi P. Systemic sclerosis. Indian F Dent Res. 2007;18(1).
2. Alpöz E, Ankaya HC and Güneri P. Facial subcutaneous calcinosis and mandibular resorption in systemic sclerosis: A case report. Dentomaxillofacial Radiology 2007;36:172–4.
3. Mehra A, Kumar S. Periodontal manifestations in systemic sclerosis: A Review. Issue Date: June 2008, Posted on: 6/26/2008.
4. J Cesar, S Guimarães, Boris A. Cruz. Severe digital ischemia due to systemic sclerosis successfully treated with bosentan: Case report. J Vasc Bras 2007;6(3):277–80.
5. Neville, Damm, Allen, Bouquot. Oral and Maxillofacial Pathology. 2nd ed, Dermatologic diseases.
6. Shafer-Hine L. Textbook of oral pathology, 5th ed.

CHAPTER 6

CREST Syndrome (Acrosclerosis)

INTRODUCTION

CREST syndrome is an uncommon condition that may be a relatively mild variant of systemic sclerosis. The term **CREST** is an acronym for **C**alcinosis cutis, **R**aynaud's phenomenon, **E**sophageal dysfunction, **S**clerodactyly and **T**elangiectasia.

CLINICAL FEATURES

As with systemic sclerosis, most patients with CREST syndrome are women in the 6th or 7th decade of life. The characteristic signs may not appear synchronously but instead may develop sequentially over a period of months to years.[1]

Calcinosis cutis occurs in the form of movable, nontender, subcutaneous nodules, 0.5–2.0 cm in size, which are usually multiple (Fig. 6.1).

Raynaud's phenomenon may be observed when a person's hands or feet are exposed to cold temperatures. The initial clinical sign is a dramatic blanching of the digits, which appear dead-white in color as a result of severe vasospasm. A few minutes later, the affected extremity takes on a bluish color because of venous stasis. After warming, increased blood flow results in a dusky-red hue with the return of hyperemic blood flow. This may be accompanied by varying degrees of throbbing pain (Fig. 6.2).

Esophageal dysfunction, caused by abnormal collagen deposition in the esophageal submucosa, may not be noticeable in the early phases of CREST syndrome. Often the subtle initial signs of this problem must be demonstrated by barium swallow radiologic studies.

The *Sclerodactyly* of CREST syndrome is rather remarkable. The fingers become stiff, and the skin takes on a smooth, shiny appearance. Often the fingers undergo permanent flexure, resulting in a characteristic "claw" deformity (Fig. 6.3). As with systemic sclerosis, this change is due to abnormal deposition of collagen within the dermis in these areas.

The telangiectasias in this syndrome are similar to those seen in hereditary hemorrhagic telangiectasia. As with that condition, significant bleeding from the superficial dilated capillaries may occur. The facial skin and vermillion zone of the lips are commonly affected (Fig. 6.4).

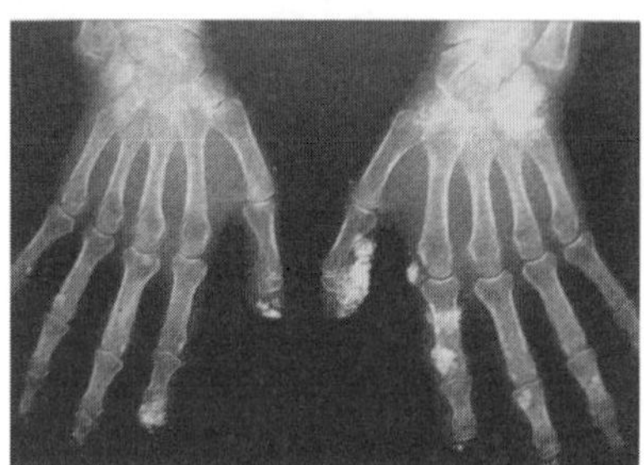

Fig. 6.1: The 'C' in CREST syndrome refers to Calcinosis, which is most frequently seen in the tendon sheaths of the fingers and within the finger pads

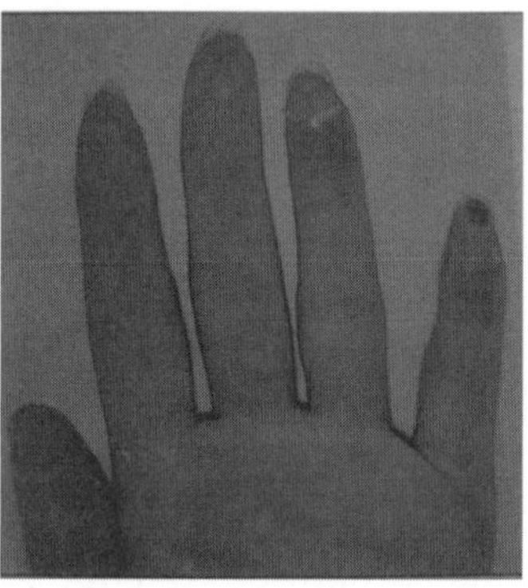

Fig. 6.2: The 'R' in CREST syndrome refers to Raynaud's phenomenon, a vasoactive response to cold that produces red, white, and blue features in the hands and fingers (referred to as patriotic sign)

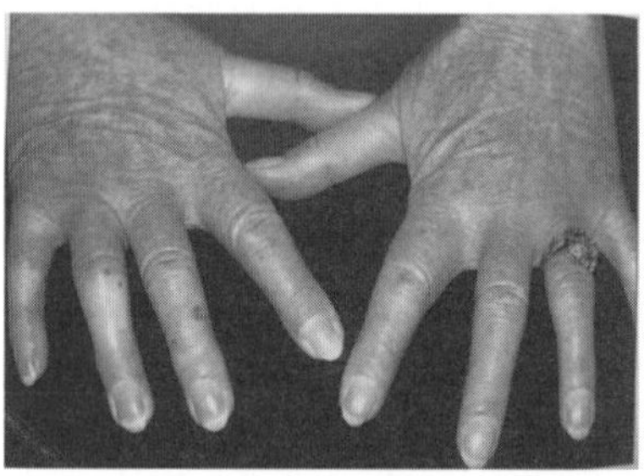

Fig. 6.3: The 'S' in CREST syndrome refers to Sclerodactyly, which is characterized by thin pointed fingers with circumferentially tight skin

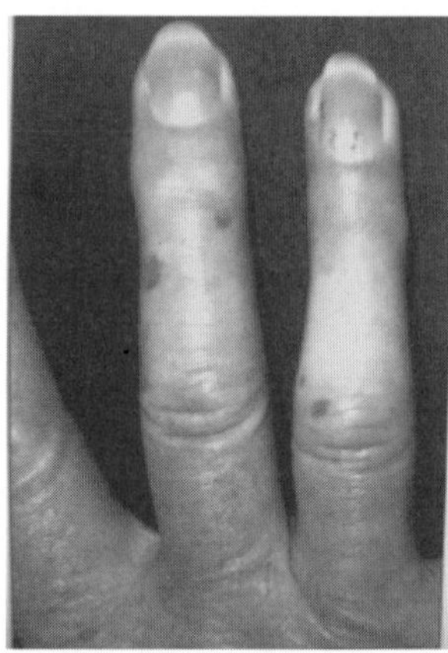

Fig. 6.4: The 'T' in CREST syndrome refers to Telangiectasia, which are most commonly seen on the tight skin of the fingers

DIAGNOSIS

Sometimes hereditary hemorrhagic telangiectasia may be considered in the differential diagnosis if the history is unclear and the other signs of CREST are not yet evident. In these cases, laboratory studies directed at identifying anticentromere antibodies may be useful, because this test is relatively specific for CREST.

HISTOLOGIC FEATURES

The histopathologic findings in CREST syndrome are similar, although milder, to those seen in systemic sclerosis. Superficial dilated capillaries are observed if a telangiectatic vessel is included in the biopsy specimen.

TREATMENT AND PROGNOSIS

The treatment of patients with CREST syndrome is essentially the same as that of those with systemic sclerosis. Because CREST syndrome usually is not as severe, the treatment does not have to be as aggressive. The prognosis is much better than for systemic sclerosis, with 80% of these patients surviving 6 years after diagnosis and 50% alive after 12 years.

REFERENCE

1. Neville, Damm, Allen, Bouquot. Oral and Maxillofacial Pathology. 2nd ed, Dermatologic diseases.

CHAPTER 7

Psoriasis

INTRODUCTION[1]

Psoriasis is a common dermatologic disease. It can occur at any age but usually first develops during young adult life and may persist throughout a person's lifetime with periods of exacerbation and remission.

ETIOPATHOGENESIS

The cause of psoriasis is unknown but it appears to be an immunoregulatory disorder in which epidermal changes are related to a defect in the control of keratinocyte proliferation, leading to a very rapid turn over rate of skin epithelial cells that is upto eight times greater than normal. A strong hereditary influence also has been suggested, particularly in the form of multifactorial inheritance.[2]

Patients do not have a genetic predisposition for the disease; the disease has a strong association with HLA Cw6 and B57 region. Recent evidence suggests that in addition to these regions many other gene loci such as 19p13, 17q25, and 1q21 may also increase the susceptibility to this disease.[3]

Triggering factors such as anxiety, stress, systemic infections, metabolic disturbances and endocrine dysfunction may increase the severity of the disease or cause an acute exacerbation.[2]

CLINICAL FEATURES[2]

Psoriasis is a chronic inflammatory dermatologic disease that may persist throughout life with periods of exacerbation and remission. The basic skin lesion of the condition is a well-defined erythematous papule or plaque covered by silver scales. Removal of the scales results in small pinpoint bleeding because of increased vascularity under focal areas of epidermal thinning. This feature occurs only in psoriasis and is known as Auspitz sign. The cutaneous lesions are often roughly symmetrical, with the majority occurring on the extensor surfaces of the extremities, scalp, back, chest, face and abdomen (Figs 7.1 and 7.2).

ORAL MANIFESTATIONS[2]

Although psoriasis is a common dermatologic disease, it rarely has been reported to manifest in oral mucous membrane lesions, Sklavounou and Laskaris reviewed the literature and found 68 reported cases until 1990.

Oral lesions may vary in type from red plaques to white plaques to ulcers (Fig. 7.3). Geographic tongue also has been listed as an oral manifestation of psoriasis but this may be a coincidental finding. A marked degree of diffuse erythema has been frequently found in patients with acute exacerbations.

Psoriasis with exclusive oral involvement also has been described, however, it is highly doubtful that oral lesions can exist without skin lesions. Therefore, diagnosis of oral psoriasis is dependent upon confirmation of concurrent cutaneous disease and is based on the patient's history, clinical examination and characteristic microscopic features.

HISTOLOGIC FEATURES[1]

The microscopic appearance of psoriasis varies with lesion age and activity. The early lesion shows parakeratosis and acanthosis with budding at the tips of the rete ridges and thinning of the suprapapillary plate. Polymorphonuclear leukocytes migrate through the epithelium with the formation of intraepithelial microabscesses. Although the formation of microabscesses (Munro abscesses) is characteristic of psoriasis, it is not specific to the disease nor are the microabscesses always present. Within the connective tissue papilla, engorgement of the capillaries occurs and a mixed inflammatory cell infiltrate is commonly seen (Fig. 7.4). In the oral cavity, this microscopic presentation, known as psoriasiform mucositis, is shared by psoriasis, Reiter's syndrome (a disease of unknown origin characterized by the triad of urethritis, arthritis and conjunctivitis), benign migratory glossitis (also known as geographic tongue) and erythema migrans (lesions that are clinically and histologically similar to geographic tongue but involve oral mucosa other than the dorsum of the tongue).

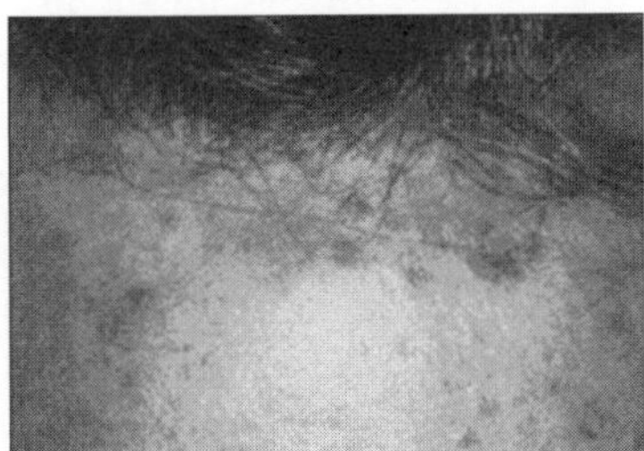

Fig. 7.1: Psoriatic lesions on the patient's scalp. The patient's cutaneous lesions presented as silvery scales

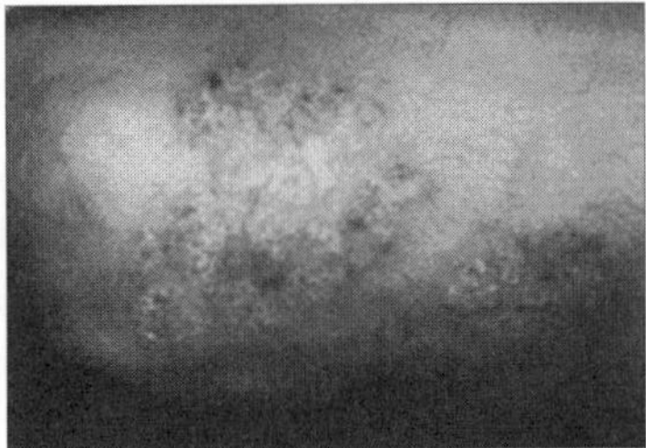

Fig. 7.2: Psoriatic lesions on the patient's elbow

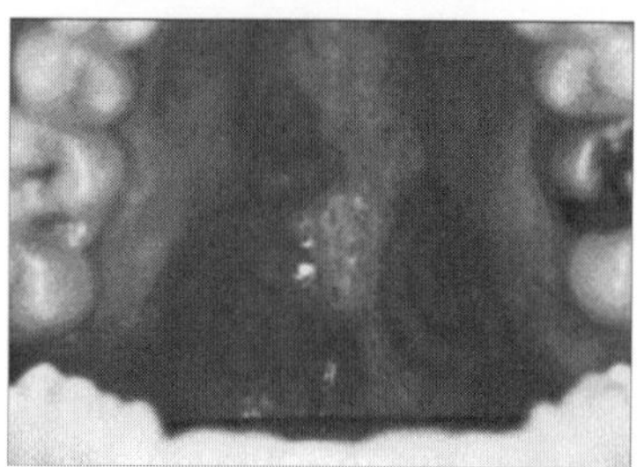

Fig. 7.3: Clinical presentation of the patient's palate. The intraoral psoriasis presented as red serpiginous linear lesions on the posterior half of the hard palate

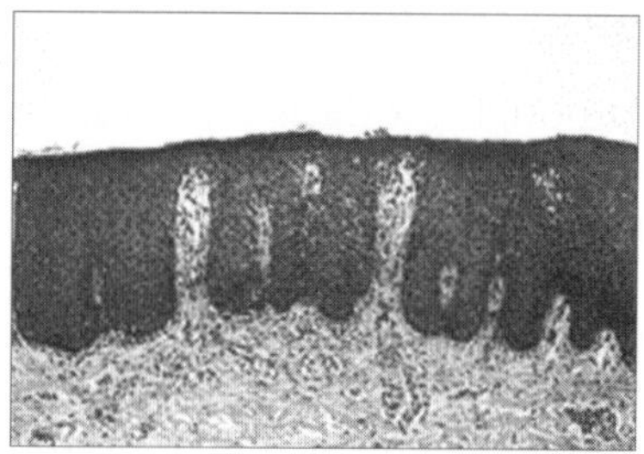

Fig. 7.4: Test-tube shaped rete ridges, thinning of the suprapapillary plate and engorgement of the capillaries in the connective tissue papilla

DIFFERENTIAL DIAGNOSIS[2]

Differential diagnosis must include 'psoriasiform' and other lesions of the oral mucosa such as Reiter's syndrome, lichen planus, eczema, syphilis, geographic tongue, candidiasis and leukoplakia.

TREATMENT[3]

The lesions are usually benign but a few cases may be refractory to treatment. Treatments for more general or advanced psoriasis include UV-A light, psoralen plus UV-A light (PUVA), retinoids (e.g. Isotretinoin, Acitretin), Methotrexate (particularly for arthritis), Cyclosporine, and Alefacept.

PROGNOSIS[2]

The prognosis of psoriasis varies from grave to excellent and improves greatly when the lesions are treated early. Spontaneous remissions occur in about 20% of all cases. Although not considered a premalignant lesion, sporadic carcinomatous changes in psoriatic lesions have been reported.

REFERENCES

1. Lisa J, Richardson F, Kratochvil J, Monica B. Zieper. Unusual palatal presentation of oral psoriasis. Journal de l'Association dentaire canadienne Février 2000,Vol;66:2.
2. Dimitrakopoulos I, Lazaridis N, Scordalak A. Dermal psoriasis involving an oral split-skin graft. Case report. Dent J 1998;43(5): 321–3.
3. Shafer-Hine L. Textbook of Oral Pathology, 5th ed.

CHAPTER 8

Pemphigus

INTRODUCTION[1]

The word Pemphigus is derived from Greek word Pemphix meaning bubble/blister for a group of potentially life-threatening autoimmune mucocutaneous diseases characterized by epithelial blistering affecting cutaneous and/or mucosal surfaces. Pemphigus affects 0.1–0.5 patients per 100000 populations per year.

Pemphigus affects the skin and oral mucosa and may also affect the mucosae of the nose, conjunctivae, genitals, esophagus, pharynx and larynx and is found mainly in middle-aged and elderly patients. There is damage to desmosomes by antibodies directed against the extracellular domains of the cadherin-type epithelial cell adhesion molecules—the desmogleins (Dsg), with immune deposits intraepithelially, and loss of cell-cell contact (acantholysis), leading to intraepithelial vesiculation.

EPITHELIAL BIOLOGY[2]

Individual cells of the skin and mucosa, the keratinocytes, are anchored to one another and to the underlying connective tissue by a number of adhesive mechanisms that secure tissue integrity, resist mechanical trauma, prevent micro-organisms from entering into the body, and protect from fluid loss. Epithelial cell-to-cell adhesion above the basal keratinocyte layer (i.e. intraepithelial cell adhesion) is secured by specific adhesion complexes known as desmosomes. In pemphigus patients, an autoimmune process disrupts desmosome function, leading to a breakdown of cutaneous and mucosal barriers. Characteristic is the presence of autoantibodies (lgG or IgA) against structural components of desmosomes resulting in epithelial cell separation (acantholysis) . This process is clinically evident as intraepithelial blister formation, hence the term "Pemphigus," derived from the Greek word *Pemphix* (bubble or blister). Research investigating epithelial blistering diseases led to the classification of more than 10 different disease types and subtypes currently categorized in the pemphigus group. Of these, oral lesions are commonly seen in pemphigus vulgaris (PV), in paraneoplastic pemphigus (PNP), and in cases of pemphigus associated with inflammatory bowel disease. PV and PNP warrant particular knowledge among dental professionals because the mucosal membranes are frequently involvement, even in early stages of disease. Recent evidence indicates that there are 2 phenotypes of PV, mucosal-dominant and mucocutaneous, with possible shifting from one to the other overtime (Figs 8.1 and 8.2).

PEMPHIGUS AND VARIANTS[1]

There are several variants of pemphigus described (Table 8.1, Flowcharts 8.1 and 8.2) with different autoantibody profiles and clinical manifestations. Typically an individual patient develops a single variant of pemphigus, although cases have been described of transition to another variant (Ishii, et al. 2000), presumably through epitope spreading (intermolecular), and the clinical manifestations of a single variant can change overtime, as discussed below. This change may be related to changes in the proportions of Dsg1 and Dsg3 autoantibodies (Harman, et al. 2001).

Table 8.1: Main types of pemphigus with oral involvement

Variant	*Localization of Ags*	*Main antigens (Ags)*	*Antibody class*	*Oral lesions*
PV localized to mucosae (Mucosal)	Desmosomes	Dsg3	IgG	Common
PV also involving skin/other mucosae (Muco-cutaneous)	Desmosomes	Dsg3 Dsg1	IgG	Common
Pemphigus foliaceus	Desmosomes	Dsg1	IgG	Uncommon
Drug-induced pemphigus	Desmosomes	Dsg3	IgG	Common
IgA pemphigus	Desmosomes	Dsg3	IgA	Uncommon
Paraneo-plastic pemphigus	Desmosomes or Hemidesmosomes	Desmocollin 1 Desmocollin 2 Desmoplakin 1 Desmoplakin 2 BP 230 Periplakin	IgG or IgA	Common

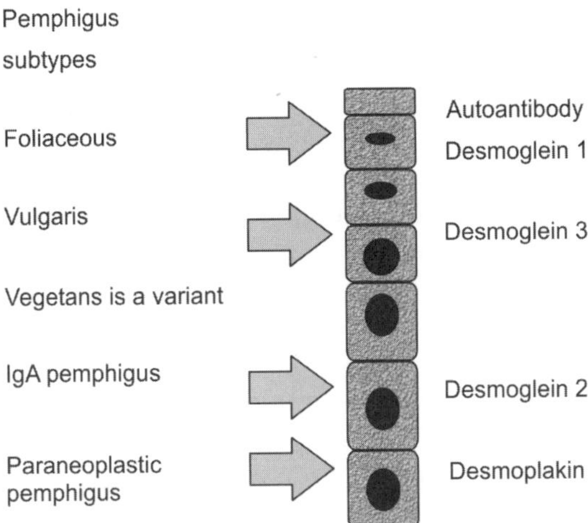

Flowchart 8.1: Variants of pemphigus

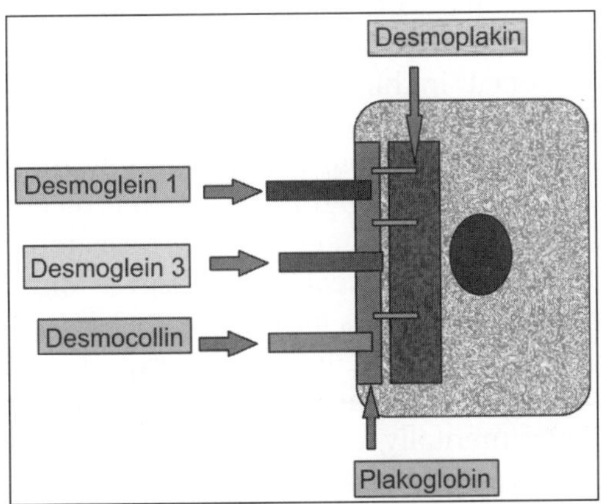

Fig. 8.1: Graphic presentation of desmosome structure:[3] Desmosomes are adhesion proteins that function both as an adhesive complex and as a cell-surface attachment site for the keratin intermediate filaments of the cytoskeleton. Desmosomes contain a series of proteins, particularly desmogleins and desmocollins—glycoproteins of the cadherin supergene family which link to cytokeratins via desmoplakins and plakoglobin (Buxton and Magee, 1992)

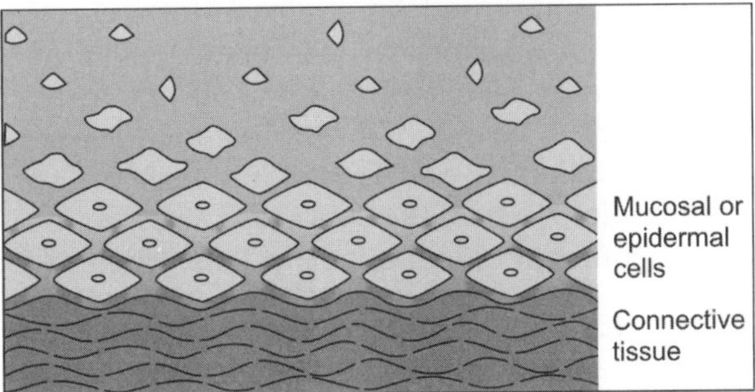

Fig. 8.2: Acantholysis

PEMPHIGUS VULGARIS

Pemphigus vulgaris (PV) is the most common form and it frequently affects the mouth (Weinberg, et al. 1997; Scully, et al. 1999). The main importance of PV is that it typically runs a chronic course, almost invariably causing blisters, erosions and ulcers on the oral mucosae and skin and, before the introduction of corticosteroids, was often fatal mainly from dehydration or secondary systemic infections (Ahmed and Moy, 1982; Robinson, et al. 1997; Scully, et al. 1999).[1]

Pathogenesis[2]

The origin of PV is unknown, but compelling evidence exists that the epithelial breakdown in PV is mediated by autoantibodies of the IgG type.

This understanding stems from passive transfer experiments in which purified autoantibodies from PV patient sera were shown to induce blisters in skin-organ culture as well as in the skin and mucous membranes of neonatal mice. When, on the other hand, the pathogenic autoantibodies were absorbed out from the patients' sera, bullae were no longer formed in the mice. Blisters occur in the epidermis and the mucous membranes, where the IgG autoantibodies target two structural proteins of the desmosomes identified as desmoglein 1 (Dsg1) and desmoglein 3 (Dsg3). A new pemphigus antigen, desmoglein 4 (Dsg4), has recently been discovered and implicated in the pathogenesis of PV. Research into the regional distribution of Dsg1 and Dsg3 revealed that Dsg1 is found throughout all layers of the skin, whereas Dsg3 is found only in 2 or 3 layers of the deep epidermis. In contrast, Dsg3 is predominantly expressed throughout mucous membranes (such as the oral epithelium), where Dsg1 is only minimally present. Experimentally, animals can be genetically engineered so that they lack Dsg3 in skin and mucous membranes (so-called "Dsg3 knockout mice"). These mice develop acantholysis like lesions in the oral mucosa but not in the skin, thus providing strong evidence that Dsg3 is of primary importance in maintaining cell attachment of mucosal surfaces. The binding of antibody to various desmogleins may have a direct effect on desmosomal adherence or may trigger a cellular process that results in acantholysis (Flowchart 8.2).

These experimental findings form the basis for an understanding of the clinical presentation. Specifically, it has been documented that some patients develop mucosal lesions without skin blisters, a phenotype of PV that has been categorized as mucosal-dominant PV. The serum of these patients contains high titers of anti-Dsg3 antibodies and low or no titers of anti-Dsgl antibodies. Hence, the preserved function of Dsg1 in the skin prevents development of cutaneous lesions, whereas the impaired adhesive function of Dsg3 causes acantholysis in the oral cavity; as PV progresses, many but not all patients develop cutaneous disease.

Cutaneous lesions appear when antibodies to both Dsg1 and Dsg3 develop, and the clinical picture of mucocutaneous PV emerges. The

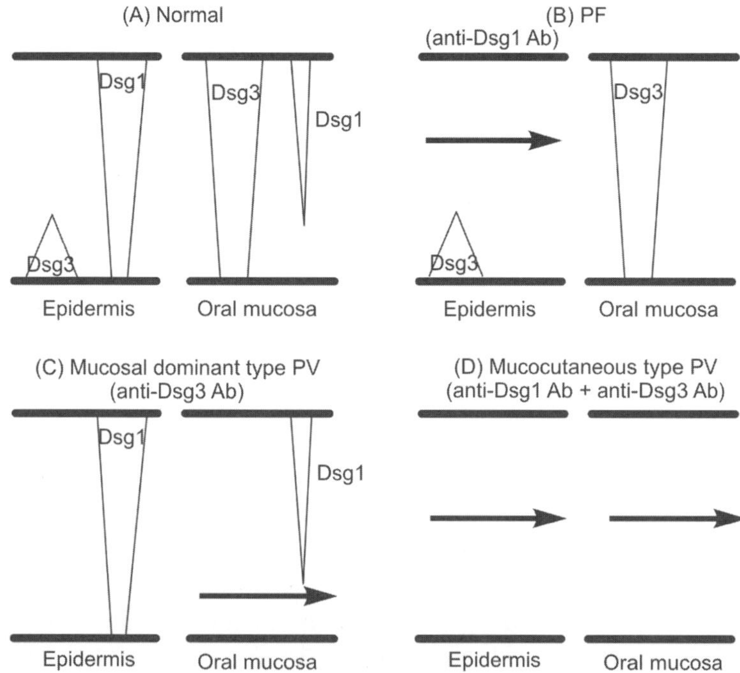

Flowchart 8.2: The distribution of Dsg1 and Dsg3 varies among epidermis and oral mucosa depending on the types of antibody (Ab) present. (A) Normal distribution. (B) Blisters occur in skin with anti-Dsg1 Ab, resulting in pemphigus foliaceus (PF). (C) Blisters occur in mucosa with anti-Dsg3 Ab, resulting in mucosal-dominant pemphigus vulgaris (PV). (D) Blisters occur in skin and mucosa with anti-Dsg1 and anti-Dsg3 Ab, resulting in mucocutaneous pemphigus vulgaris (PV). Arrows indicate the levels of blister formation. From Hashimoto T. Recent advances in the study of the pathophysiology of pemphigus

clinical phenotype thus seems to be determined by the relative amounts of antibodies against Dsgl and Dsg3. On rare occasions, anti-Dsg3 antibodies may disappear from the serum while anti-Dsgl antibodies persist. The "then-emerging" condition is pemphigus foliaceus, a pemphigus variant characterized by skin blisters without mucous membrane involvement. The observation that mucosal-dominant PV commonly precedes mucocutaneous PV puts the dentist in the forefront of diagnostic responsibility.

Besides IgG antibodies found in PV, IgA antibodies against Dsg3 also have been identified. It is rare, however, to find oral lesions in IgA pemphigus (H. Hashimoto, personal communication, February 2004), possibly because autoantigens for IgA pemphigus may in fact not be a component of desmosomes or because anti-Dsg autoantibodies may not act alone to cause pemphigus. The traditional concept of pemphigus pathophysiology as described previously is being debated, and other autoantibodies that accompany antibodies directed against Dsgl and Dsg3 may also play pivotal roles in the development of pemphigus.

What initiates the formation of IgG autoantibodies in PV patients at the very beginning of the disease is currently unknown (as is the case for most autoimmune diseases), although loss of tolerance for autoimmune target molecules may play a key role. Exogenous factors capable of inducing or perpetuating pemphigus in genetically predisposed individuals include various medications, dietary components, and environmental factors.

POSSIBLE ETIOLOGIC FACTORS[1]

- *Diet*

  Garlic may cause occasional cases of pemphigus and this and other dietary factors.
- *Drugs*

  Drugs capable of inducing pemphigus fall into 2 main groups according to their chemical structure—
  - Drugs containing a sulfhydryl radical (thiol drugs or SH drugs), e.g. Penicillamine and Captopril.
  - Nonthiol drugs, often sharing an active amide group in their molecule, e.g. Phenol drugs, Rifampicin, Diclofenac, and other ACE inhibitors are occasionally implicated.
- *Viruses*

  The apparently transmissible nature of some pemphigus variants, has suggested a role for viruses. The onset of PV has occasionally been reported concurrently with, or following, herpes virus infections, and the possibility of epitope spreading or molecular mimicry have been suggested as the pathogenesis. Herpes virus DNA has been detected in peripheral blood mononuclear cells and skin lesions of patients with pemphigus by PCR. Human herpes virus 8 (HHV-8) DNA was detected in lesions of patients with PV compared with nonpemphigus blistering skin diseases which were negative but HHV-8 might have trophism for pemphigus lesions. Indeed, others have failed to detect HHV-8 DNA in lesional skin of patients with PV.
- *Other factors*

  A recent multicenter study at outpatient services of teaching hospitals in Bulgaria, Brazil, India, Israel, Italy, Spain and the USA revealed lower numbers of smokers among patients with PV, higher exposure rates to pesticides, and a higher number of female patients who had been pregnant and suggested that this may point to the contribution of estrogens in the disease process.
- *Association with other disorders*

  Pemphigus vulgaris may occasionally be associated with other autoimmune disorders such as rheumatoid arthritis, myasthenia gravis, lupus erythematosus, or pernicious anemia.
- Certain HLA haplotypes (A10 or A26, DRW6) are thought to be associated, suggesting a genetic predisposition.

- It has been reported more frequently in certain racial groups for example the Ashkenazi Jews and those of Mediterranean descent.

CLINICAL FEATURES[4]

The initial manifestations of pemphigus vulgaris often involve the oral mucosa, typically in adults. The average age at diagnosis is 50 years, although rare cases may be seen in childhood. No sex predilection is observed, and the condition seems to be more common in Jews.

Patients usually complain of oral soreness, and examination shows superficial ragged erosions and ulcerations distributed haphazardly on the oral mucosa, buccal mucosa, ventral tongue, and gingivae are often involved (Figs 8.3 and 8.4). Patients rarely report vesicles or bullae formation intraorally, and such lesions can seldom be identified by the examining clinician, probably because of early rupture of the thin, friable roof of the blisters. Over 50% of the patients have oral mucosal lesions before the onset of cutaneous lesions, sometimes by as much as 1 year or more. Eventually, however, nearly all patients have intraoral involvement. The skin lesions appear as flaccid vesicles and bullae that rupture quickly, usually within hours to a few days, leaving an erythematous, denuded surface. Infrequently ocular involvement may be seen, usually appearing as bilateral conjunctivitis. Unlike cicatricial pemphigoid, the ocular lesions of pemphigus do not tend to produce scarring and symblepharon formation.

Without proper treatment, the oral and cutaneous lesions tend to persist and progressively involve more surface area. A characteristic feature of pemphigus vulgaris is that a bulla can be induced on normal-appearing skin if firm lateral pressure is exerted. This is called a *positive Nikolsky sign.*

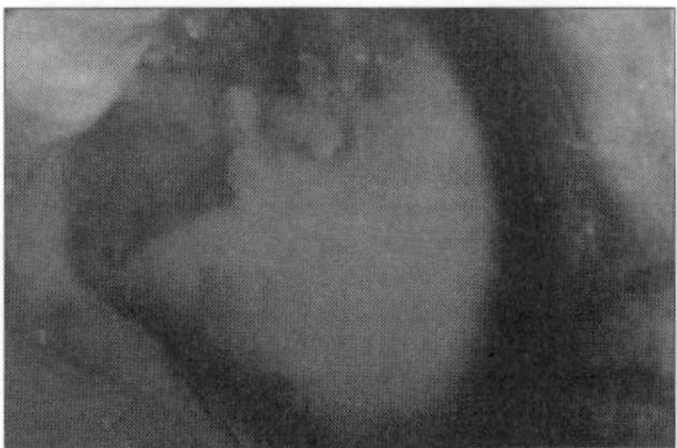

Fig. 8.3: Multiple erosion of the buccal mucosa

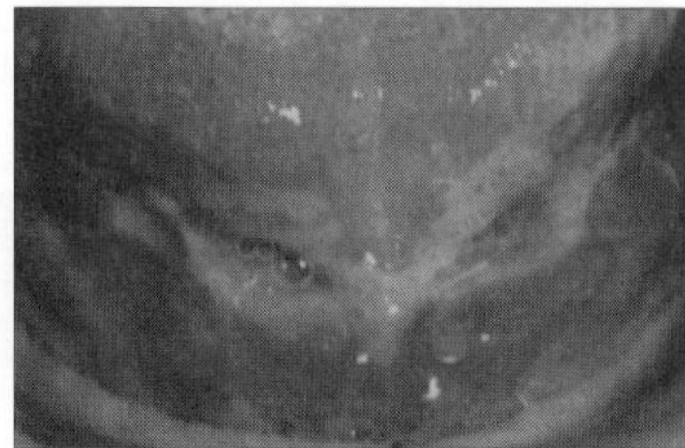

Fig. 8.4: Large irregular-shaped ulcerations involving floor of the mouth and ventral tongue

HISTOLOGIC FEATURES[4]

Biopsy specimens of perilesional tissue show characteristic intraepithelial separation, which occurs just above the basal cell layer of the epithelium. Sometimes the entire superficial layers of the epithelium are stripped away, leaving only the basal cells, which have been described as resembling a "row of tombstones". The cells of the spinous layer of the surface epithelium typically appear to fall apart, a feature that has been termed acantholysis, and the loose cells tend to assume a rounded-shape. This feature of pemphigus vulgaris can be used in making a diagnosis based on the identification of these rounded cells (Tzanck cells) in an exfoliative cytologic preparation. A mild-to-moderate chronic inflammatory cell infiltrate is usually seen in the underlying connective tissue (Figs 8.5 and 8.6).

The diagnosis of pemphigus vulgaris should be confirmed by direct immunofluorescence examination of fresh perilesional tissue or tissue submitted in Michel's solution. With this procedure, antibodies (usually IgG or IgM) and complement components (usually C3) can be demonstrated in the intercellular spaces between the epithelial cells in almost all patients with this disease. Indirect immunofluorescence is also typically positive in 80%–90% of cases, demonstrating the presence of circulating autoantibodies in the patient's serum (Fig. 8.7).

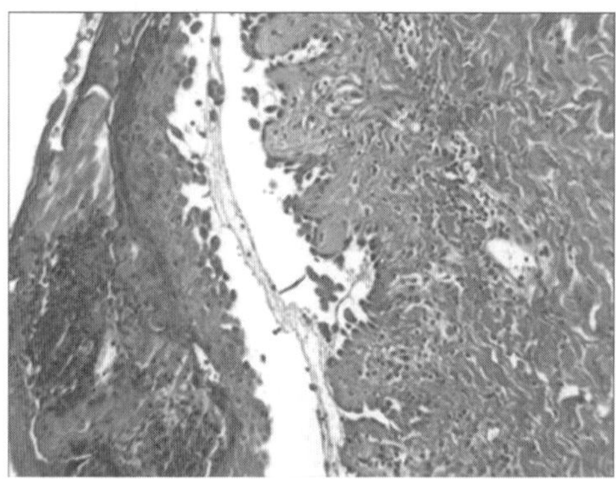

Fig. 8.5: Acantholysis: Loss of cell cohesion in the superficial layers of mucoepidermal tissue

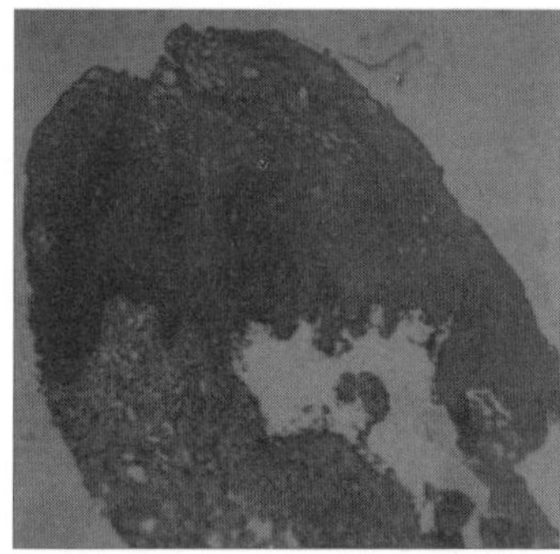

Fig. 8.6: Microscopy showing the intraepithelial cleft above the basal cell layer

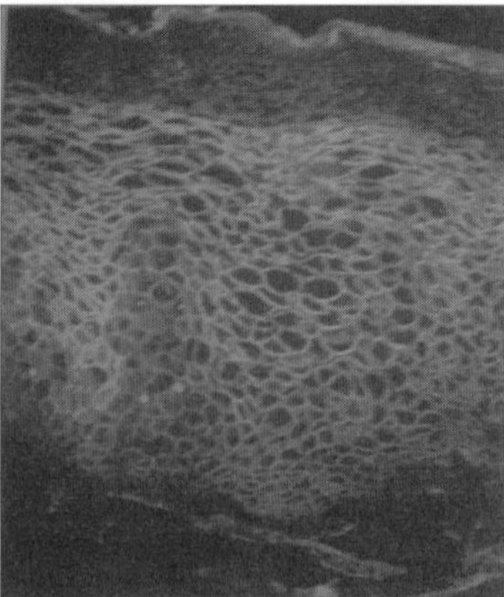

Fig. 8.7: DI showing intracellular deposition of IgG

It is critical that perilesional tissue be obtained for both light microscopy and direct immunofluorescence to maximize the probability of a diagnostic sample.

If ulcerated mucosa is submitted for testing, the results are often inconclusive because of either a lack of an intact interface between the epithelium and connective tissue or a great deal of nonspecific inflammation.

TREATMENT AND PROGNOSIS[4]

A diagnosis of pemphigus vulgaris should be made as early in its course as possible because control is generally easier to achieve. Pemphigus is a systemic disease; therefore, treatment consists primarily of systemic corticosteroids (usually Prednisolone), often in combination with other immunosuppressive drugs (so-called "steroid-sparing" agents), such as Azathioprine. Although some clinicians have used topical corticosteroids in the management of oral lesions, the observed improvement is undoubtedly because of the absorption of the topical agents, resulting in a greater systemic dose. The potential side effects associated with the long-term use of systemic corticosteroids are significant and include:

- Diabetes mellitus
- Adrenal suppression
- Weight gain
- Osteoporosis
- Peptic ulcer
- Severe mood swings
- Increased susceptibility to a wide range of infections.

Ideally, a physician with expertise in immunosuppressive therapy should manage the patient. The most common approach is to use relatively high doses of systemic corticosteroids initially to clear the lesions, and then attempt to maintain the patient on as low a dose of corticosteroids as it is necessary to control the condition. Often the success of therapy can be monitored by measuring the titers of circulating autoantibodies using indirect immunofluorescence, because disease activity often correlates with the abnormal antibody levels. Pemphigus rarely undergoes complete resolution although remissions and exacerbations are common.

Before the development of corticosteroid therapy, as many as 60% to 80% of these patients died, primarily as a result of infections and electrolyte imbalances. Even today, mortality rate associated with pemphigus vulgaris is in the range of 5%–10%, usually because of the complications of long-term systemic corticosteroid use.

REFERENCES

1. Black M, Mignogna MD, Scully C. Mucosal diseases series. Pemphigus vulgaris. Oral Diseases 2005;11(2):119–30.
2. Dominik A Ettlin. Pemphigus. Dent Clin N Am 2005;49:107–25.
3. Scully C, Bagan JV, Black M. Mucosal diseases series, epithelial biology. Oral Diseases 2005;11(1):58–71.
4. Neville, Damm, Allen, Bouquot. Oral and Maxillofacial Pathology, 2nd ed, Dermatologic diseases.

CHAPTER 9 Paraneoplastic Pemphigus

INTRODUCTION

Paraneoplastic pemphigus (PNP) is an autoimmune mucocutaneous disease frequently associated with lymphoproliferative disorders. The rare combination of the disease with other malignancies such as different types of carcinomas, sarcomas, melanoma and skin tumors has also been reported.[1] PNP was first described by Anhalt, et al. (1990)[2] as a clinically and immunologically distinct disease and proposed a set of criteria in order to arrive at the diagnosis. He initially suggested 5 criteria for the diagnosis of PNP.

1. Mucocutaneous blistering and ulcerations.
2. Histopathological features such as acantholytic changes of the epithelium and epidermis with interface dermatitis.
3. Deposition of immunoglobulin (Ig)G and C3 in intercellular areas and/or along the basement membrane.
4. Presence of serum antibodies.
5. Demonstration of various desmoplakins and desmogleins in the serum.

Recently presented 4 revised minimal criteria for diagnosis of PNP:

1. Painful, progressive stomatitis, with preferential involvement of the tongue. This finding is so consistent that it is unreasonable to consider the diagnosis in its absence.
2. Histologic features of acantholysis or lichenoid or interface dermatitis. Although acantholysis is most readily detected in oral lesions, the necrosis and secondary inflammation make it difficult to detect without repeated biopsies. Some patients never develop skin lesions; some show only lesions that clinically and histologically are lichenoid or resemble erythema multiforme. direct immunofluresence (DIF) frequently is negative, and the serologic markers for the disease are so specific that demonstration of tissue bound autoantibodies is not an essential criterion.
3. Demonstration of antiplakin autoantibodies. These auto-antibodies are the key serologic markers for the entity. Positive

indirect immunofluresence (IIF) on rodent bladder is readily available but is not highly reliable. Immunochemical techniques are much more precise and should demonstrate, at a minimum, autoantibodies against periplakin and/or envoplakin. Patients with PNP should have a positive IIF test on monkey esophagus and have antibodies against Dsg3 by ELISA. This test does not discriminate between pemphigus vulgaris (PV) and pemphigus foliaceus (PF), however.

4. Demonstration of an underlying lymphoproliferative neoplasm. Approximately two-thirds of cases arise in the context of known malignant disease, most often non-Hodgkin's lymphoma or chronic lymphocytic leukemia. In approximately one-third of cases, there is no known neoplastic lesion at the time the mucocutaneous disease develops. These cases tend to be associated with Castleman's disease, abdominal lymphoma, thymoma, or retroperitoneal sarcomas. In most cases, the occult neoplastic lesion can be detected by CT scan of the chest, abdomen, and pelvis.

Most patients develop very severe oral ulceration and conjunctival ulceration with or without genital ulceration resembling the features of Stevens-Johnson syndrome or most severe forms of drug eruption.[3] Immunopathology of PNP has been extensively studied during the last few years.[3]

CLINICAL FEATURES

Although there had been case reports of unusual pemphigus in the literature, the term PNP was proposed with sound criteria for diagnosis only in 1990 by Anhalt, et al.[2,3] The disease is of paramount importance to dental clinicians as oral ulceration is the most consistent feature of the disease (Fig. 9.1).

The age range of affected individuals may vary from 7 to 77 years.[4] Most patients exhibit very severe and painful oral ulceration. Although some patients may not develop, conjunctival ulceration appears to be a frequent feature (Fig. 9.2). The oral ulcers mimic the appearance of either severe form of erythema multiforme or severe forms of other types of drug eruptions. Genital ulceration is also a common feature. The involvement of skin in PNP shows variable appearances such as target lesions of erythema multiforme, blisters mimicking bullous pemphigoid or lichen planus like lesions.

The association of an underlying malignancy demands the necessity of correct diagnosis of PNP even quicker, as the existence of a neoplasm is recognized prior to the eruption of lesions only in about two-thirds of the cases.

Out of all the reported cases of PNP, hematologically related malignancies and disorders account for 84% and the commonest malignancy

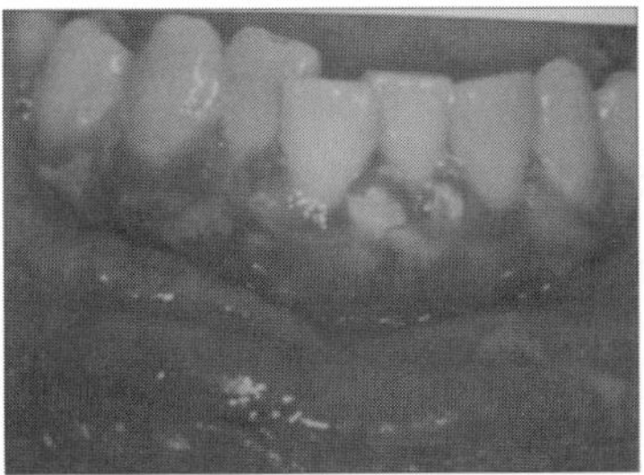

Fig. 9.1: Oral lesions in paraneoplastic pemphigus are typically vesiculobullous and very painful. Mucosal involvement is extensive. Skin lesions may also resemble lichen planus

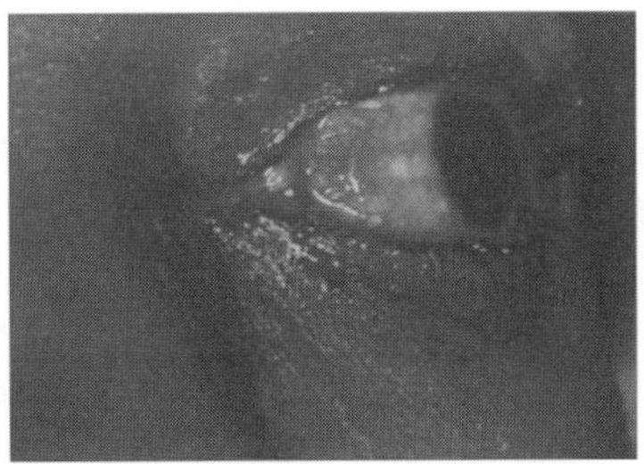

Fig. 9.2: Paraneoplastic pemphigus frequently involves the conjuctiva. Scarring may occur as in ocular pemphigoid

appears to be non-Hodgkin's lymphoma (38%).[1] Chronic lymphocytic leukemia (18%), Castleman's disease (18%), thymoma (5.5%), Waldenström's macroglobulinemia (1.2%) and Hodgkin's lymphoma (0.6%) are the other reported hematologial disorders. It is obvious that PNP can also be associated with nonhematological malignancies (16%) such as carcinomas including squamous cell carcinoma of the oral cavity, sarcomas and melanomas.[1]

PATHOGENESIS

It has been shown that proteins of plakin family and desmogleins play an important role in the pathogenesis of PNP. Truncated recombinant glutathione-S-transferase fusion proteins of envoplakin and periplakin which presented various N-terminal and C-terminal domains have shown to be very strongly reactive with sera from patients with PNP. Further, it has been showed that all the PNP antigens identified upto date belong to the plakin family.[3]

Because of the fact that plakins have cytoplasmic location, they are not directly accessible to autoantibodies in intact cells. Therefore, it is believed that the autoantibodies directed towards desmogleins (1 and 3) start the damage of cell membrane exposing the plakins. Flare-up of PNP has been reported to occur with medications to underlying malignancy such as fludarabine and interferon alpha.

DIAGNOSTIC CRITERIA

The diagnostic criteria for PNP have been proposed with the introduction of the disease by Anhalt, et al. (1990).[2] They include mucocutaneous blistering and ulcerations, histopathological features such as acantholytic changes of the epithelium and epidermis with interface dermatitis, deposition of IgG and C3 in intercellular areas and/or along the basement membrane, presence of serum antibodies and finally demonstration of various desmoplakins and desmogleins in the serum. The histopathology is different from that of conventional pemphigus by the presence of keratinocyte necrosis, less pronounced acantholytic changes and a marked interface dermatitis like cell infiltrate (Fig. 9.3). Direct immunofluorence (DIF) usually shows weak or moderate positivity in the intercellular area for IgG and C3. Some cases may show granular or linear deposits of the same at the basement membrane.

One important factor which needs to be stressed is the fact that if PNP is strongly suspected clinically, negative histology and DIF does not completely rule out the possibility of the disease.

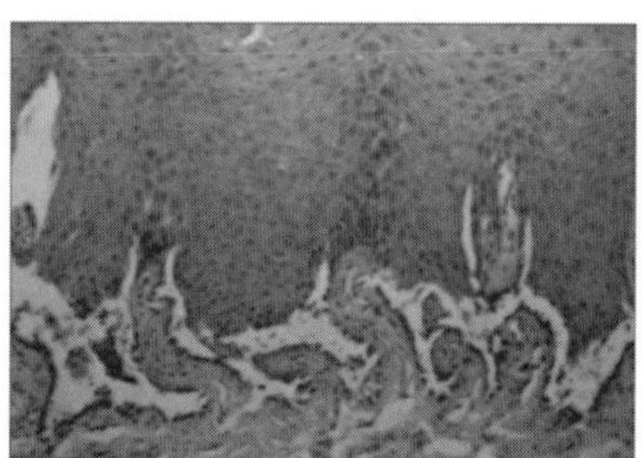

Fig. 9.3: A suprabasilar separation in a case of paraneoplastic pemphigus

TREATMENT

Although the treatment of choice for PNP is oral Prednisolone, it is frequent to use adjuvant treatment including Cyclophosphomide, Azathioprine, Cyclosporine A, Gold, Dapsone, plasmapheresis, photopheresis and various combinations of the above. However, it is not unusual to find that majority of patients become refractory to treatment.

Recently, the use of monoclonal antibodies such as anti-CD 20 antibody has also been reported to be of help in order to treat cases with the disease. The prognosis of PNP with malignant tumors is generally poor and 90% die within 2 years and the mean survival for majority of the patients is 3 months after the diagnosis.

REFERENCES

1. Kaplan I, Hodak E, Ackerman L, et al. Neoplasms associated with paraneoplastic pemphigus: A review of literature with emphasis on non-haematologic malignancy and oral manifestations. Oral oncology 2004;40: 553–62.
2. Anhalt GL, Kim SC, Stanley JR, et al. Paraneoplastic pemphigus: An autoimmune mucocutaneous disease. N Engl J Med 1990;323:1729–35.
3. Hashimoto T. Immunopathology of paraneoplastic pemphigus. Clin Dermatol 2001;19: 675–82.
4. Anhalt GL. Paraneoplastic pemphigus. Adv Dermatol 1997;12:77–96.

CHAPTER 10

Pemphigoid and Other Basement Membrane Diseases

INTRODUCTION

Mucous membrane pemphigoid (MMP) is a chronic, subepithelial autoimmune disease, which predominantly involves mucosal surfaces and results in mucosal blistering, ulceration, and subsequent scarring. The condition belongs to a group of mucocutaneous autoimmune blistering disorders often collectively referred to as subepithelial bullous dermatoses (SEBDs). These disorders result in blistering of the skin or oral mucosa and include bullous pemphigoid (BP), MMP, linear IgA disease (LAD), chronic bullous dermatosis of childhood (CBDC), and epidermolysis bullosa acquisita (EBA).[1]

It is about 50 years since pemphigoid was recognized as a clinical phenotype distinct from the previously recognized bullous diseases pemphigus and dermatitis herpetiformis (Lever, 1953). A decade later, the in vivo linear deposition of immune deposits (immunoglobulins, complement or both) along the epithelial basement membrane zone (BMZ) was recognized to characterize pemphigoid. The immune deposits at the BMZ were shown to consist predominantly of IgG and C3. Pemphigoid was then recognized actually to be a family of diseases which included conditions such as BP and pemphigoid (herpes) gestations, which generally affect the skin and have only minor oral involvement, and cicatricial pemphigoid (CP) which mainly involves the mucous membranes, most frequently the ocular and oral mucosae.[2]

A number of other subepithelial vesiculobullous disorders were subsequently recognized and the term intramembrane subepithelial bullous dermatoses (IMSEBD) was thus introduced, recognizing that the autoantibodies can be directed against antigens of the BMZ different from the classic bullous pemphigoid antigens. The BP antigen and several newly identified antigens share the feature that IgG is located on the floor of salt-split skin biopsies. The antigens include epiligrin, uncein, 105 kDa protein, 200 kDa protein, type-IV collagen, and type-VII collagen (associated with epidermolysis bullosa acquisita). Thus, the clinical entity often previously termed pemphigoid came to be recognized to include CP [now renamed mucous membrane pemphigoid, MMP], BP, pemphigoid gestations

(PG), anti-p200, anti-p105 and anti-p450 pemphigoid, lichen planus pemphigoides, dermatitis herpetiformis, linear IgA disease, EBA, bullous systemic lupus erythematosus (SLE) and paraneoplastic pemphigus (Table 10.1).[2]

Table 10.1: Autoimmune bullous skin diseases

Bullae	*Disease*
Intraepithelial	Pemphigus Pemphigus vulgaris Pemphigus vegetans Pemphigus herpetiformis Pemphigus foliaceus Endemic pemphigus (fogo selvagem) Pemphigus erythematous Drug-induced pemphigus IgA pemphigus Paraneoplastic pemphigus
Subepithelial	Pemphigoid BP PG Lichen planus pemphigoides CP MMP Ocular cicatricial pemphigoid Anti-plectin pemphigoid Anti-p105 pemphigoid Anti-p200 pemphigoid Epidermolysis bullosa acquisita Dermatitis herpetiformis Duhring Linear IgA disease

CLASSIFICATION OF PEMPHIGOID GROUP OF DISEASES[3]

Traditionally, pemphigoid group of diseases has been classified into 2 main clinical subgroups:

- Bullous pemphigoid: It usually involves skin, but 30% of the time involves oral mucous membrane.
- Cicatricial pemphigoid: This involves mucous membrane (usually oral and or conjunctival) and skin to lesser extent (20%) and with less severity.

Today, pemphigoid group has been categorized into:

1. Cicatricial pemphigoid
2. Oral mucous membrane pemphigoid
3. Ocular pemphigoid.

EPITHELIAL BIOLOGY[2]

Cell-epithelial basement membrane contact is largely, via hemidesmosomes, which link the keratinocyte cytoskeletons to the lamina lucida—the superficial part of the epithelial basement membrane (Table 10.2).

The deeper aspect of the epithelial basement membrane is the lamina densa, which is anchored to the underlying papillary dermis by cross-banded anchoring fibrils. The epithelial basement membrane and adjacent area is termed the epithelial BMZ.

The epithelium and BMZ, thus have a complex structure and an array of protein molecules is required for normal epithelial integrity. Inevitably, if anyone or more of these BMZ proteins is defective or damaged, the result can be loss of cell-basement membrane adhesion, leading to subepithelial vesiculation and the clinical phenotype of pemphigoid. The etiological agents responsible are varied and often unknown but many of the disorders damaging these molecules are of autoimmune etiology (IMSEBD), can affect several epithelia and may have systemic manifestations (Table 10.3). Rare disorders such as epidermolysis bullosa are due to gene mutations affecting these hemidesmosome associated proteins.

The clinical phenotype, which is acquired and consists of vesicles, bullae and/or erosions affecting mucosae predominantly, is termed MMP, and it is this condition, which commonly affects the mouth.

Table 10.2: Main hemidesmosome components

Protein	*Alternate terms*	*Site*	*Disease*
Keratin 5		Basal layer of stratified epithelia	Epidermolysis bullosa simplex
Keratin 14		Basal layer of stratified epithelia	Epidermolysis bullosa simplex
Plectin/HD1		Intracellular	Epidermolysis bullosa simplex with muscular dystrophy
IFAP300		Intracellular	?
P200		Intracellular	?
BPAg1	BP230 or dystonin	Intracellular	Bullous pemphigoid
BPAg2	BP180 or type-XVII collagen	Transmembrane	Cicatricial pemphigoid, bullous pemphigoid
$\alpha6\beta4$ integrin		Transmembrane	Cicatricial pemphigoid junctional epidermolysis bullosa
Laminin 5	Epiligrin or nicein or kalinin	BMZ	Cicatricial pemphigoid junctional epidermolysis bullosa
Laminin 6		BMZ	?
Ladinin	LAD-1	BMZ	?
Uncein		BMZ	?
Type-VII collagen		BMZ	Epidermolysis bullosa dystrophica, epidermolysis bullosa acquisita
Type-IV collagen		BMZ	?

Table 10.3: Subepithelial vesiculobullous disorders (immune mediated subepithelial blistering diseases

Disease	*Antigen involved*
Pemphigoid	Table 10.4
Dermatitis herpetiformis	Epidermal transglutaminase (TGas 3)
EBA	Type-VII collagen
Bullous SLE	Type-VII collagen
Toxic epidermal necrolysis	105 kDa
Linear IgA disease	45 kDa
Chronic bullous dermatosis of childhood	97 kDa

Table 10.4: Antigens implicated singly or in combination in pemphigoid variants

Disease	*Antigen*
BP	BP230 kDa mainly BP180 kDa 105 kDa antigen
MMP	BP180 kDa mainly BP230 kDa Laminin 5 Laminin 6 Uncein β4 Integrin subunit α6 Integrin subunit 200 kDa 168 kDa 45 kDa
PG	180 kDa 230 kDa

MUCOUS MEMBRANE PEMPHIGOID

Introduction[1]

MMP involvement may include the eyes, oral cavity, and pharyngeal mucosa of patients usually over the age of 50 years. Although MMP is a blistering disease predominantly involving the mucosal surfaces, upto 30% of patients may also have skin involvement. On an immunohistopathologic level, autoantibodies produced by MMP patients target one of several different autoantigens in the mucosal or epithelial basement membrane zone (BMZ). This antibody and antigen interaction causes the cleaving of fibrils in the basement membrane, as well as the activation of complement with the recruitment of neutrophils, which eventually results in subepithelial blistering.

Pathophysiology[1]

The pathophysiologic mechanism of MMP is complex and is not yet completely understood. There is clearly a defect in the immune regulation involving the formation of autoantibodies, usually of the IgG class, directed against normal components (antigens) of the BMZ. This interaction triggers a complicated web of immunologic events resulting in the expression of inflammatory mediators that induce migration of lymphocytes, eosinophils, neutrophils, and mast cells to the BMZ. The separation of epithelium from the underlying tissue within the BMZ may be the result of direct cytotoxic action or the effect of lysosomal proteolytic enzymes. Fibroblasts also are activated secondary to the production of inflammatory cytokines. The collagen produced may lead to cicatrization of the eye or mucous membranes. This process is of particular importance in MMP affecting the eyes, where fibrosis or subsequent cicatrization can cause profound tear insufficiency, symblepharon formation, trichiasis, keratinization of the cornea, and several other defects.

Clinical presentation[1]

Oral lesions occur in more than 90% of individuals with MMP, whereas oral involvement may be present in upto 50% of those with BP. Oral manifestations of MMP are variable and often include desquamative gingivitis associated with severe gingival erythema and frank ulceration. Ulceration or atrophy of the buccal and labial mucosa, palate, and tongue are also frequently observed (Fig. 10.1). An intraoral ulcer may present with a pseudomembrane consisting of a necrotic eschar covering. Intact vesicles (filled with clear fluid or blood) are rare in the oral cavity but may be observed (Fig. 10.2).

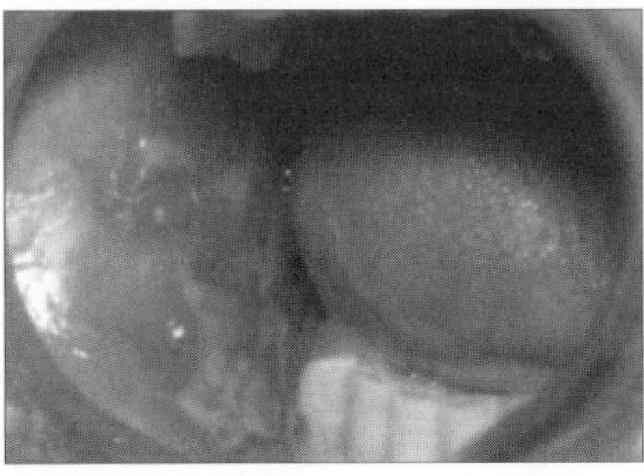

Fig. 10.1: Buccal mucosa of a patient with MMP, notice the ulceration and the scarring

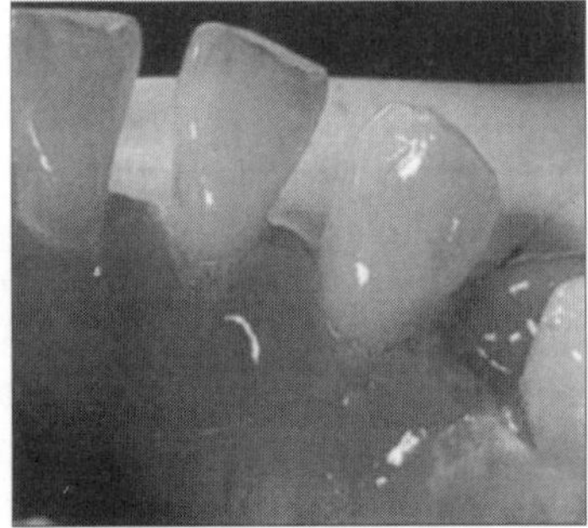

Fig.10.2: Intact blood-filled vesicle

Most patients are symptomatic, often complaining of oral pain caused by mucosal ulceration and desquamation. Patients with gingival involvement frequently have poor oral hygiene because of the inability to clean the dentition effectively secondary to mucosal pain.

Thus, patients may often present with bleeding gums. Patients typically describe the inability to eat certain types of foods for fear of exacerbating the symptoms. Occasionally patients may complain of halitosis, from lack of maintaining good oral hygiene. Other common clinical observations include delayed or incomplete healing following scaling and root planning or peeling of the gingival tissue with simple prophylaxis. Soft tissue management during dental restoration may also be compromised and associated with extensive bleeding. Consequently, impression taking and retraction cord placement can be difficult in patients with MMP.

Occasionally, the signs and symptoms of MMP may be subtle. Anecdotally, some patients may notice a superficial sloughing of the oral mucosa. Other patients may describe a transient fluid-filled blister that ulcerates and quickly heals. On the other hand, long-standing lesions related to MMP may be secondarily infected, sore and slow to heal.

Extraoral manifestations of MMP can involve the conjunctiva, genitalia, esophagus, trachea, and larynx. Involvement of the esophagus may result in dysphagia and odynophagia, whereas tracheal involvement may lead to hoarseness. Eye involvement may initially be characterized by conjunctival injection. Later, symblepharon formation may occur. Symblepharon formation results from the scarring and adhesion of the bulbar to the palpebral conjunctiva (Fig. 10.3). As a result, corneal damage is common, and progressive scarring can lead to blindness. Genital involvement results in mucosal ulceration and may lead to sexual dysfunction resulting from pain. Although MMP is considered a subepithelial blistering mucosal disorder, MMP involves the skin in upto 30% of patients. Most of the other subepithelial blistering disorders are much more likely than MMP to involve the skin and should be considered in a well-developed differential diagnosis if both the oral mucosa and skin are involved.

Histologic features[2]

The MMP is histologically characterized by junctional separation at the level of the basement membrane giving rise to a subbasilar split as in other forms of pemphigoid. Classical histopathological features include a subepithelial split with a chronic inflammatory infiltrate containing eosinophils, lymphocytes, and neutrophils as well, in the lamina propria (Fig. 10.4). However, routine biopsy of a patient suspected of having MMP is often not enough to fully differentiate the disease from other mucocutaneous disorders.

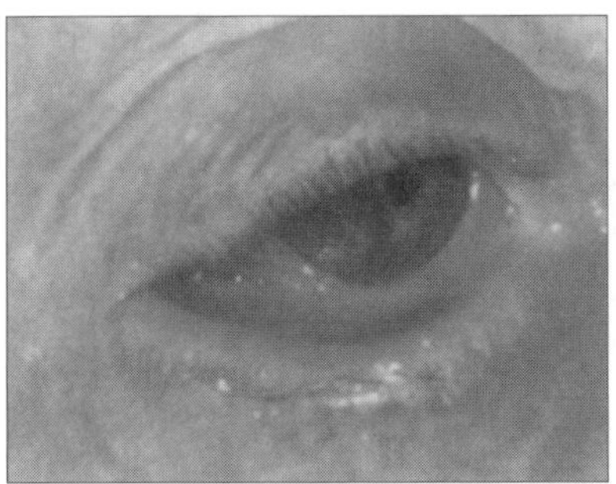

Fig.10.3: Symblepharon formation resulting from the scarring of the bulbar and palpebral conjunctiva

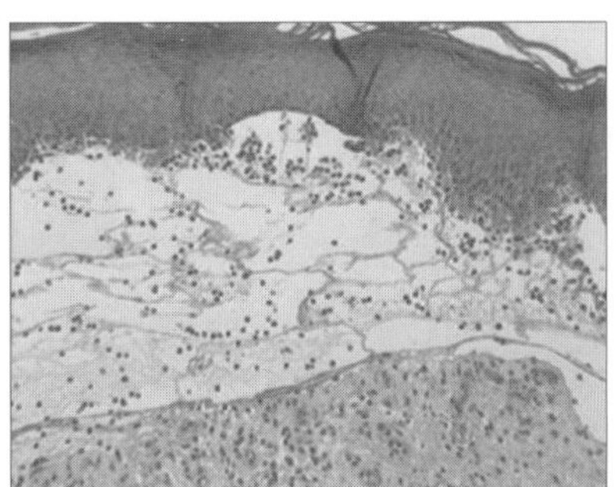

Fig. 10.4: Histological aspects of a bulla in a case of OMMP

DIRECT IMMUNOFLUORESCENCE (DIF)[2]

Essentially all patients with MMP and CP have, on DIF, in vivo bound IgG, IgA or C3, presenting as a homogeneous line in the BMZ of lesional and perilesional mucosa (Figs 10.5A and B). Deposition of C3 in the BMZ is detected in almost all patients, sometimes is the sole immunologic reactant, and is considered diagnostically significant. The DIF analysis of biopsy specimens of MMP where the epithelium is separated from the underlying connective tissue may show IgG deposits on the basal pole of the epithelial cells in an interrupted linear pattern.

DIF is, thus, useful in several ways: First, a positive result confirms the diagnosis of IMSEBD. Second, DIF differentiates IgG-mediated diseases [BP, MMP, HG and acquired epidermolysis bullosa (EBA)] from IgA mediated diseases (dermatitis herpetiformis and linear IgA disease).

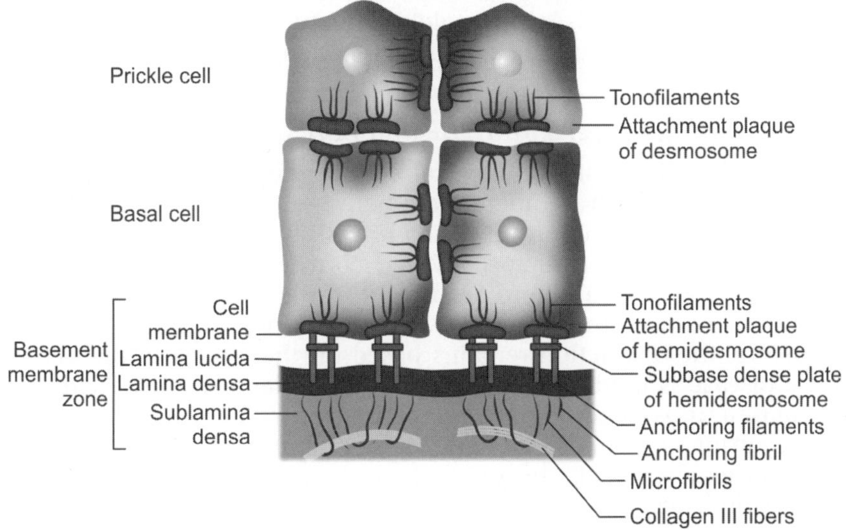

Fig. 10.5A: Stratified squamous epithelium and the basement membrane zone

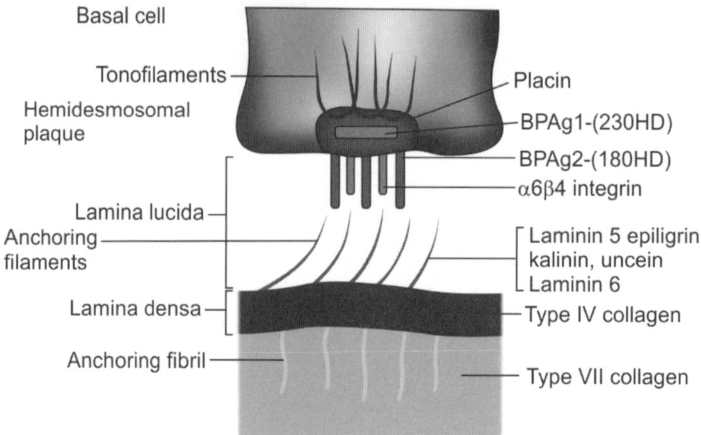

Fig. 10.5B: The hemidesmosomes and the basement membrane zone

Diagnosis[2]

The differential diagnoses of MMP may include pemphigus vulgaris, and bullous SLE as well as pemphigoid subtypes and other IMSEBD. The management can only be carried out appropriately if there is an accurate diagnosis, and this is based on the history, examination, and biopsy with histological and direct immunofluorescent (DIF) examination.

Routine histopathology of a properly obtained specimen will demonstrate subbasilar cleavage. The most appropriate area to biopsy is not an erosion, which will show loss of the epithelium one wishes to study, but a vesicle or perilesional tissue. Some suggest inducing a vesicle by rubbing the mucosa first before taking a biopsy.

It is better to avoid gingival biopsy since the chronic inflammation of gingivitis may confuse the histological picture. Also obtaining a diagnostic gingival biopsy can be technically challenging and result in a periodontal defect.

Differentiating between MMP, BP and EBA

Even after routine histopathological and immunopathological studies, it can still be difficult to differentiate between MMP, BP and EBA. Oral lesions are more common MMP than in BP but are indistinguishable clinically and by light microscopy and conventional immunostaining though eosinophils are more prominent in BP. The MMP and BP may be differentiated ultrastructurally, but this is not routinely available. Therefore, the distinction remains based on the clinical presentation; if the disease is predominantly cutaneous, a diagnosis of BP is made, whereas if it is predominantly mucosal, specially when associated with scarring, a diagnosis of MMP is more appropriate. The EBA may also present clinical, histopathological and immunopathological features indistinguishable from MMP. In doubtful cases, the very best distinction can be achieved by using human skin split in 1 M sodium chloride through the lamina lucida prior to IIF examination. If immune deposits are limited to the floor (dermal side) of the induced cleavage, the diagnosis is most likely to be EBA, whereas if deposits are also on the roof side, the diagnosis is MMP.

If the serum does not contain detectable antibodies, concentrated serum should be used. If these results are negative, 2 other tests can be performed.

1. A split may be induced chemically in intact perilesional tissue for DIF examination in a way similar to IIF, when epidermal and dermal fluorescence indicates MMP (Gammon, et al. 1990).
2. A definitive diagnosis may be obtained determining the antigen-binding specificity of circulating antibodies using immunoblotting or immunoprecipitation (Mutasim, 1997). EBA sera, unlike MMP, label the 290 kDa major component and a minor 145 kDa protein from dermal extracts.

Management[2] (Flowchart 10.1)

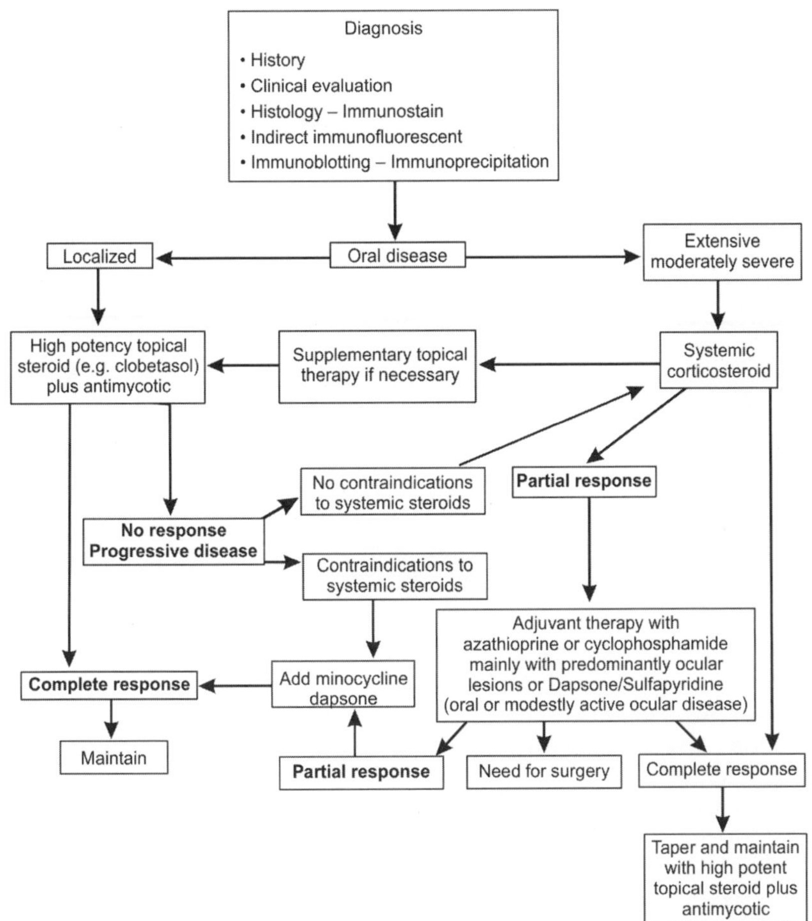

Flowchart 10.1: Management of pemphigoid and other basement membrane disease

REFERENCES

1. Sollecito Thomas P, Parisi E. Mucous membrane pemphigoid. Dent Clin N Am 2005;49:91–106.
2. Bagan J, Muzio LL, Scully C. Mucosal diseases series. Mucous membrane pemphigoid. Oral Diseases 2005;11(3):197–218.
3. Marx R. Oral and Maxillofacial Pathology.

CHAPTER 11

Erythema Multiforme

(Synonyms: Lyell's syndrome, Stevens-Johnson syndrome, toxic epidermal necrolysis)

INTRODUCTION

Erythema multiforme (EM) is an acute mucocutaneous hypersensitivity reaction characterized by a skin eruption, with or without oral or other mucous membrane lesions. Occasionally, EM may involve the mouth alone. EM has been classified into a number of different variants based on the degree of mucosal involvement and the nature and distribution of the skin lesions. EM minor typically affects no more than one mucosa, is the most common form and may be associated with symmetrical target lesions on the extremities. EM major is more severe, typically involving two or more mucous membranes with more variable skin involvement which is used to distinguish it from Stevens-Johnson syndrome (SJS), where there is extensive skin involvement and significant morbidity and a mortality rate of 5–15%. Both EM major and SJS can involve internal organs and typically are associated with systemic symptoms. Toxic epidermal necrolysis (TEN) may be a severe manifestation of EM, but some experts regard it as a discrete disease. EM can be triggered by a number of factors, but the best documented is preceding infection with herpes simplex virus (HSV), the lesions resulting from a cell-mediated immune reaction triggered by HSV–DNA. SJS and TEN are usually initiated by drugs, and the tissue damage is mediated by soluble factors including Fas and FasL.

EM is an uncommon, acute inflammatory disorder, which affects the skin and/or mucous membranes. There is a spectrum of clinical presentations encompassed under the diagnosis, described below.

Erythema multiforme is a reactive mucocutaneous disorder that comprises variants ranging from a self-limited, mild, exanthematous, cutaneous variant with minimal oral involvement (EM minor) to a progressive, fulminating, severe variant with extensive mucocutaneous epithelial necrosis SJS and TEN. All variants share 2 common features: Typical or less typical cutaneous target lesions and satellite cell or more widespread necrosis of the epithelium. These features are considered to be sequelae of a cytotoxic immunologic attack on keratinocytes expressing nonself-antigens. These antigens are primarily microbial (viruses) or drugs. (Ayangco and Rogers, 2003). However, there are significant differences in severity and clinical expression between EM minor, EM major, SJS and TEN.

Erythema multiforme usually affects apparently healthy young adults and several reports suggest that males are affected more than females. The peak age at presentation is between 20 and 40 years although 20% of cases occur in children. The disease is often recurrent and is precipitated by preceding herpes infection in upto 70% of cases (Carrozzo, et al. 1999).

Etiology

A range of usually exogenous factors trigger what appears to be an immunologically related reaction with sub and intraepithelial vesiculation.

- There may be a genetic predisposition to EM, with associations of recurrent EM with HLA-B15 (B62), HLA-B35, HLA-A33, HLA-DR53 and HLA- DQB1*0301. HLA DQ3 has been proven to be specially related to recurrent EM and may be a helpful marker for distinguishing herpes-associated EM (HAEM) from other diseases with EM-like lesions.
- Patients with extensive mucosal involvement may have the rare HLA allele DQB1*0402.
- Erythema multiforme has been reported to be triggered by numerous agents, particularly viruses, specially HSV but other herpes viruses (varicellazoster virus, cytomegalovirus, Epstein-Barr virus), adenoviruses, enteroviruses (Coxsackievirus B5, echoviruses), hepatitis viruses (A, B and C), influenza, paravaccinia, parvovirus B19, poliomyelitis, vaccinia and variola have all been implicated.
- A variety of other infectious agents, which are less commonly implicated, may include bacteria such as *Mycoplasma pneumoniae*, borreliosis, cat scratch disease, diphtheria, hemolytic streptococci, legionellosis, leprosy, *Neisseria meningitidis*, *Mycobacterium avium* complex, pneumococcus, proteus, pseudomonas, rickettsia, salmonella, staphylococcus, syphilis, tuberculosis, tularemia, typhoid, *Vibrio parahemolyticus*, yersinia, chlamydia, *Lymphogranuloma venereum* and psittacosis, fungal infections such as coccidioidomycosis, dermatophytes or histoplasmosis and parasites such as Trichomonas and *Toxoplasma gondii*.
- Immune conditions such as BCG or hepatitis B immunization, sarcoidosis, graft-versus-host disease, inflammatory bowel disease,

polyarteritis nodosa or systemic lupus erythematosus may be implicated (Ayangco and Rogers, 2003).

- Food additives or chemicals such as benzoates, nitrobenzene, perfumes or terpenes have also been reported as etiological agents.
- Drugs such as sulfonamides (e.g. cotrimoxazole), cephalosporins, aminopenicillins, quinolones, chlormezanone, barbiturates, oxicam nonsteroidal anti-inflammatory drugs, anticonvulsants, protease inhibitors, allopurinol or even corticosteroids may be implicated (Porter and Scully, 2000; Diz Dios and Scully, 2002; Abdollahi and Radfar, 2003; Scully and Bagan, 2004). In one series, antecedent medication use was identified in 59% of EM patients and 68% of SJS patients, and a striking increase in the number of cases in one series caused by cephalosporins (Stewart, et al. 1994). In general there appears to be an association between the type of etiological agent and the severity of the disease. Thus, viral infections appear to trigger EM minor or major but drug ingestion tends to trigger more severe SJS or TEN. However, this is not absolute and a small but significant proportion of EM minor and major cases are precipitated by drugs, while likewise some cases of SJS are virally associated (Auquier-Dunant, et al. 2002).
- The etiology of EM is unclear in most patients, but appears to be an immunological hypersensitivity reaction with the appearance of cytotoxic effector cells, CD8+ T lymphocytes, in epithelium, inducing apoptosis of scattered keratinocytes and leading to satellite cell necrosis (Ayangco and Rogers, 2003).

Herpes associated erythema multiforme (HAEM)

The best documented association is between HSV infection and EM minor/major and has been designated as HAEM. Evidence that EM may be triggered by HSV has come from a number of sources.

In single episode and recurrent EM many patients give a history of a preceding herpes infection 2 weeks or less before onset of the disease (Leigh, et al. 1985; Nesbit and Gobetti, 1986; Huff and Weston, 1989; Farthing, et al. 1995) and the antiviral agent acyclovir is successful in treating a high proportion of patients with recurrent EM (Molin, 1987; Huff, 1988; Tatnall, et al. 1995) even when there is no clear clinical association with HSV infection (Lozada and Silverman, 1978). A number of studies have sought HSV or HSV–DNA in lesions of EM. Infectious HSV has not been recovered from the lesions (Kokuba, et al. 1998) but HSV–DNA has been detected in 36–81% (Brice, et al. 1989; Darragh, et al. 1991; Aslanzadeh, et al. 1992; Miura, et al. 1992; Imafuku, et al. 1997; Kokuba, et al. 1999). The large variation in detection rates may be due in part to differences in the selection criteria for cases included for analysis but it seems clear that detection of lesional HSV–DNA is not restricted to those cases showing a clinical association with HSV. One study looked at HSV–

DNA expression in single episode and recurrent HAEM (documented to be related to HSV infection) as well as idiopathic EM not associated with either preceding HSV infection or drug ingestion (Ng, et al. 2003) and found that similar proportions of lesions (upto 60%) were positive for HSV–DNA in both groups. This together with the observation that antiviral drugs are successful in treating some patients with recurrent lesions without a clinical association of HSV suggests that some cases of idiopathic EM may actually be related to a subclinical HSV infection or reactivation.

Little is known about the HSV genotype in relation to HAEM. One study found that the lip was the most common site of preceding HSV infection in recurrent EM implicating HSV-1 (Farthing, et al. 1995). A more recent study using nested PCR found HSV-1 in 66%, HSV-2 in 28% and both HSV-1 and HSV-2 in 6% of the patients (Sun, et al. 2003).

Histology

Lesions of EM are similar histopathologically both in the oral mucosa and the skin. They are characterized by a lichenoid infiltrate in the basement membrane zone of the epidermis or epithelium. T lymphocytes and mononuclear cells are present in the dermis and lamina propria and extend into the epithelium or epidermis obscuring the basement membrane zone. The degree of mononuclear cell infiltration is variable and tends to be less in those lesions resembling TEN. The epithelium or epidermis may appear edematous and spongiotic and there is necrosis both of basal and suprabasal epithelial cells, resulting in both intra and subepithelial bullae formation. Not infrequently the bullae contain mononuclear cells (Fig. 11.1). Immunofluorescence shows granular staining for C3 at the basement membrane zone and occasionally within vessels or apoptotic keratinocytes (Ayangco and Rogers, 2003).

In cases resembling TEN, there is prominent epidermal damage but with little inflammatory infiltration either within the epidermis or in the dermis.

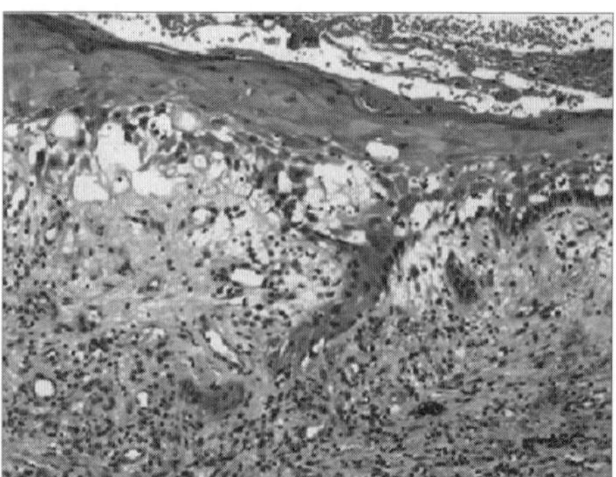

Fig. 11.1: Histopathology of EM minor. The epithelium is edematous and intra- and subepithelial vesicles are present. An infiltration of lymphocytes and macrophages is seen in the lamina propria and within the epithelium

Pathogenesis

Erythema multiforme appears to be the result of a cell-mediated immune reaction to the precipitating agent. In HAEM, it is most likely that HSV–DNA fragments in the skin or mucosa precipitate the disease. HSV–DNA fragments and in particular DNA polymerase (PoL) have been detected in the basal and suprabasal cell layers of the epidermis in lesions as well as healed lesions for upto 3 months (Imafuku, et al. 1997) and the T cells accumulating in active lesions are CD4+ (Vb2+) cells which respond to HSV antigens in vitro (Malmstrom, et al. 1990; Kokuba, et al. 1998). In addition, there is a good correlation between PoL expression in lesions, CD4+ (Vb2+) T cell accumulation and the duration of clinical symptoms (Kokuba, et al. 1998). In situ RT-PCR and immunocytochemical staining have shown that mononuclear cells in both HAEM and HSV lesional skin tissues stain positively for IFN-c, a cytokine, which is associated with tissue damage, and this expression correlates with HSV-protein expression (Kokuba, et al. 1999). IFN-c is produced by CD4+ T helper 1 (Th1) lymphocytes, cells characteristic of a delayed type hypersensitivity reaction (DTH) (Billiau, et al. 1998) (Fig. 11.2). IFN-c is proinflammatory and induces adhesion molecule expression on keratinocytes and endothelial cells as well as stimulating production of chemokines and cytokines from a number of cell types. Thus, it seems likely that the HSV–DNA fragments in skin or mucosa initiate a specific T-cell mediated DTH response resulting in the presence of HSV-specific T cells, which generate IFN-c. This cytokine then amplifies the immune response and stimulates the production of additional cytokines and chemokines, which aids the recruitment of further reactive T cells to the area. These cytotoxic T cells, NK cells or chemokines can all induce epithelial damage.[1]

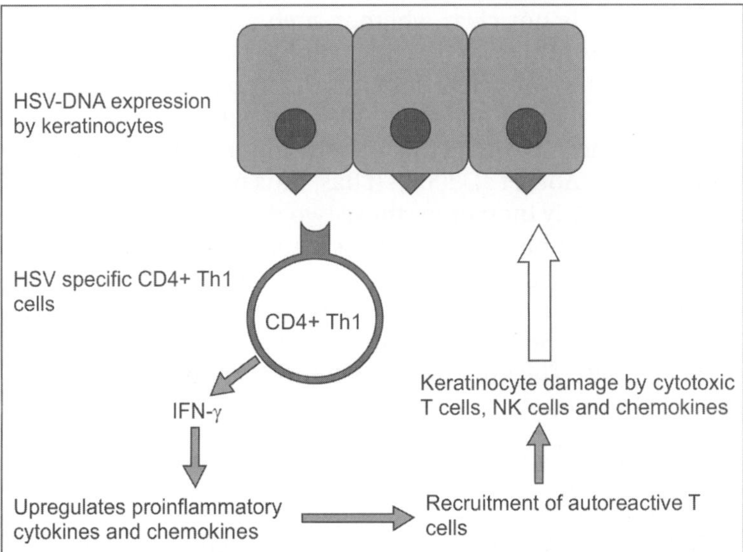

Fig. 11.2: Pathogenesis of erythema multiforme

The mechanisms of tissue damage in EM appear to differ between virally induced and drug-induced EM and also differ from those in SJS and TEN, particularly those that are characterized by widespread epithelial damage but with a sparse inflammatory infiltrate. For example, in drug-induced EM, it is thought that reactive metabolites of the initiating drug induce the disease (Knowles, et al. 2000) but the mechanisms of damage are variable and unlike HAEM do not appear to be the result of a DTH response. Immunocytochemicial staining and in situ hybridization has shown that T cells do not produce IFN-γ in drug-induced lesions but rather the lesions are characterized by tumor necrosis factor alpha (TNF-α) present in keratinocytes and also produced by macrophages and monocytes. In contrast, TNF-α has not been detected in HAEM and it has even been proposed that its presence may be used as a laboratory test to distinguish drug-induced lesions from HAEM (Aurelian, et al. 2003). Much of the tissue damage in drug-induced lesions appears to be due to apoptosis and, because of the paucity of the inflammatory reaction; attention has recently been focused on soluble factors and cytokines. Locally produced TNF-α may be important since, it has been shown to mediate keratinocyte apoptosis (Paul, et al. 1996) and it is possible this mechanism plays a role in milder forms of drug-induced EM.

However, particularly in TEN and SJS, there is some evidence for a Fas–FasL interaction. FasL mediates apoptotic cell death by binding to Fas on cells and inducing the formation of caspases. Fas is present on keratinocytes (Sayama, et al. 1994) and FasL is found on activated T cells and NK cells (Iwai, et al. 1994) and thus binding of keratinocytes to T cells or NK cells can induce apoptosis.

One report suggests that keratinocytes in TEN may express FasL, which could potentially induce cell death in a neighboring keratinocyte (Viard, et al. 1998) but it is not clear whether such a mechanism is generally operative. There is also evidence that soluble FasL (sFasL) produced by peripheral blood mononuclear cells may be important, since high levels of sFasL are present in the peripheral blood of patients with SJS and TEN, and sera from these patients are able to induce marked keratinocyte apoptosis in vitro (Abe, et al. 2003). It has, thus been proposed that sFasL levels may be an early marker for these two diseases.

In addition to soluble factors, there is some evidence that keratinocyte cell death may be mediated directly by cytotoxic T cells since lymphocytes isolated from the blister fluid of a patient with TEN were cytotoxic towards autologous cells only in the presence of the precipitating drug (Nassif, et al. 2002). The apoptotic mechanism appeared to be mediated by perforin/granzyme.

Clinical Features

Erythema multiforme may present a wide spectrum of severity, from mild limited disease to a severe, widespread and life-threatening illness (Ayangco and Rogers, 2003). Skin lesions are usually symmetrical and consist of macules or erythematous papules, which develop into classical target or iris lesions. Occasionally, bullae may be seen.

Skin lesions are often accompanied by ulceration of mucous membranes particularly the oral cavity. Head and neck manifestations were present in 4 of 79 patients (5%) with EM and 26 of 28 patients (93%) with SJS in one series (Stewart, et al. 1994). In SJS, mucosal involvement of the lip (93%), conjunctiva (82%), oral cavity (79%) and nose (36%) were most common.

Most patients with EM (70%) of either minor or major forms have oral lesions (Fig. 11.3). Oral involvement may precede lesions on other stratified squamous epithelia, or may arise in isolation. It typically presents with;

- Lesions that progress through diffuse and widespread macules to blisters and ulceration
- Lips that become swollen and cracked, bleeding and crusted
- Intraoral lesions typically on the nonkeratinized mucosae and most pronounced in the anterior parts of the mouth.

Recurrences are seen in about 25%; the periodicity can vary from weeks to years; usually attacks last for 10–20 days once or twice a year and usually resolve after about 6 episodes (range: 2–24) within a mean period of 10 years (range: 2–36 years).

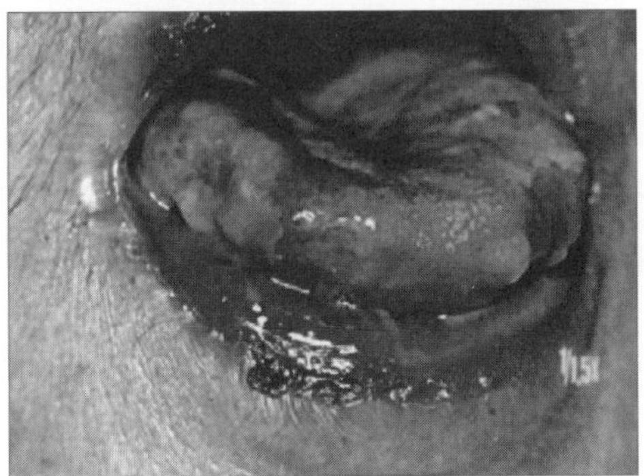

Fig. 11.3: Clinical appearance of EM

Skin lesions

Skin lesions have been classified as [(Bastuji-Garin, et al. 1993) and these have been used to subclassify EM]

1. **Typical targets**: They are defined as individual lesions less than 3 cm diameter with a regular round shape, a well-defined border, and two concentric palpable, edematous rings, paler than the center disc. These lesions are most common in EM minor and milder forms of EM major in a symmetrical distribution on the extensor surfaces of the extremities.
2. **Raised atypical targets**: It appears similar to target lesions and are palpable erythematous lesions with a rounded shape but poorly

defined borders and a dark central area, which may erode and become necrotic. These lesions are most common in severe EM major or in SJS.
3. **Flat atypical targets**: As their name suggests are not palpable and they form ill-defined erythematous areas with a tendency to central blister formation. These lesions are most common in SJS.
4. **Erythematous or purpuric macules with or without blister formation**: They are of variable size and may become confluent. These lesions are most common in SJS and TEN.

Other mucosae

- Eye involvement may cause lacrimation and photophobia (Fig. 11.4).
- Genital lesions are painful and may result in urinary retention (Fig. 11.5).

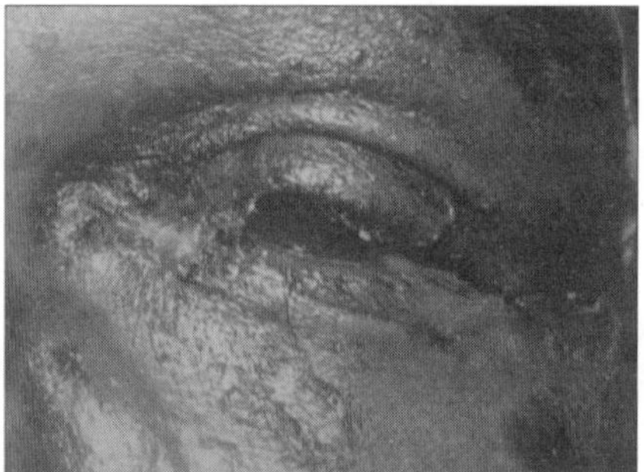

Fig. 11.4: The ocular lesions of erythema multiforme major are corneas and conjunctiva necrosis along with some skin necrosis

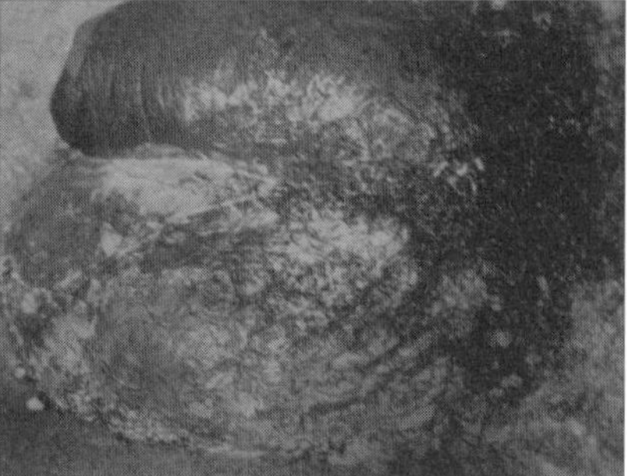

Fig. 11.5: The genital lesions of erythema multiforme major are skin necroses of the scrotum and penis. One percent silver sulfadiazine is used here as an antimicrobial cream similar to burn wound management

Clinical Variants

Erythema multiforme has been subdivided into different clinical types based on the severity of the presentation. Originally, the disease was classified as either EM minor or major (Huff, et al. 1983) and distinction between the two depended principally on the extent of mucosal involvement. SJS was considered to be a severe variant of EM major. Then TEN was added to the disease spectrum (Lyell, 1993) and confusion arose over the diagnostic criteria for the different subtypes.

A consensus paper (Bastuji-Garin, et al. 1993) has defined the more severe clinical variants based on morphology of the skin lesions, their extent and distribution and the extent of epidermal detachment, as bullous EM, SJS, SJS/TEN overlap, TEN with spots with or without blisters and TEN without spots but it remains to be determined whether each represents distinct etiopathological entities.

Erythema Multiforme Minor

Erythema multiforme minor is considered the mildest form of EM and is characterized by skin lesions, which are usually symmetrically distributed on the extensor surfaces of the arms and legs. Rashes are various but typically are '**iris or target**' lesions or bullae on extremities (Fig. 11.6). The lesions may be itchy and accompanied by systemic symptoms such as fever and malaise (Ayangco and Rogers, 2003). By definition, mucous membrane involvement is limited to only one site and usually, it is the oral mucosa alone that is affected (Huff, et al. 1983).

Occasionally, lesions may occur orally prior to their appearance on the skin or sometimes only the oral cavity is affected. Intraoral lesions occur predominantly on the nonkeratinized mucosa and are most pronounced in the anterior parts of the mouth. The lips are also commonly affected and are swollen and cracked, bleeding and crusted (Fig. 11.7). Typically, oral lesions progress through diffuse widespread macules to blisters and ulceration although only ulceration may be seen at presentation. In these cases, diagnosis may be difficult.

Although considered by some to be a benign self-limiting disease, some cases of recurrent EM minor may be very severe, particularly if accompanied by widespread oral ulceration (Farthing, et al. 1995). In these cases the lips tend to be spared.

Erythema Multiforme Major

Erythema multiforme major is characterized by involvement of multiple mucous membranes (Huff, et al. 1983). Generally, EM major is a more severe form of the disease than EM minor and, in addition to the ocular, genital, oral cavity, the genital, ocular, laryngeal and esophageal mucosa may be affected (Figs 11.4, 11.5, 11.8a, 11.8b). The skin lesions, however,

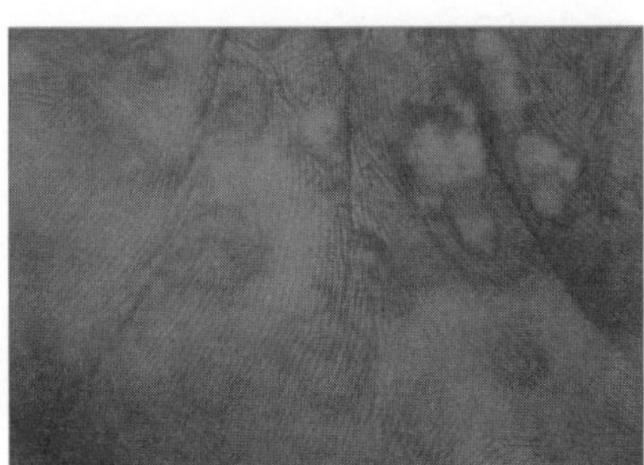

Fig. 11.6: "Classic" erythema multiforme skin lesions will appear t:arget-like and are best seen on the palms of the hands

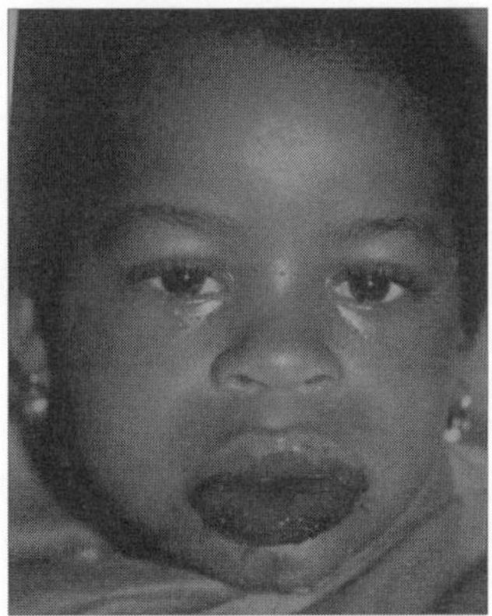

Fig. 11.7: Erythema multiforme minor has severe pain and a fast onset. Here a 5-year old developed three target skin lesions and a painful lower lip lesion within hours after taking the antibiotic cefaclor

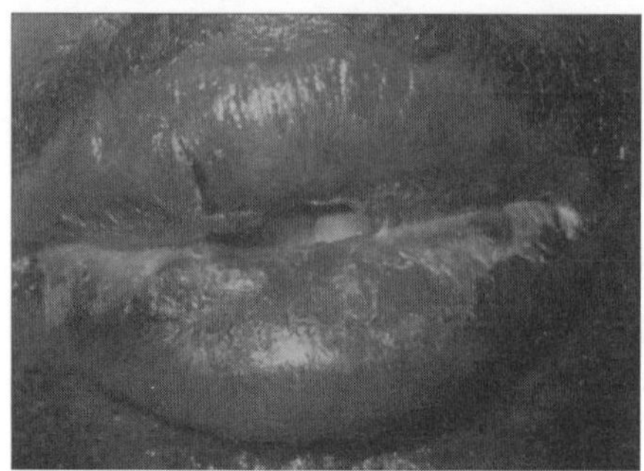

Fig. 11.8a: Early onset of erythema multiforme major with beginning erosive surface lesions of the vermillions

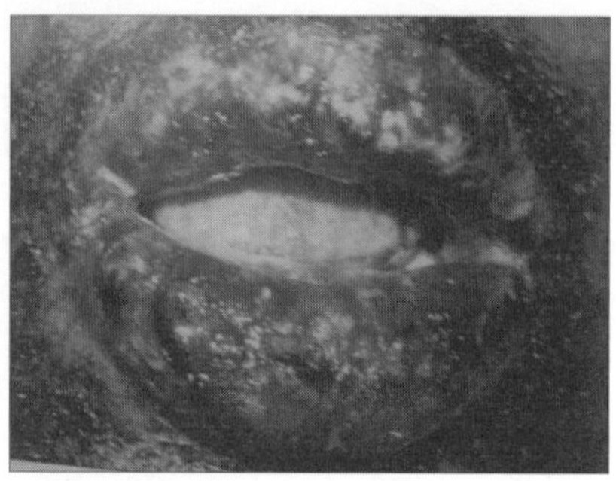

Fig. 11.8b: Within 24 hours, the beginning erosions have necrosed the entire vermillion surface to create a painful hemorrhagic crusting lip

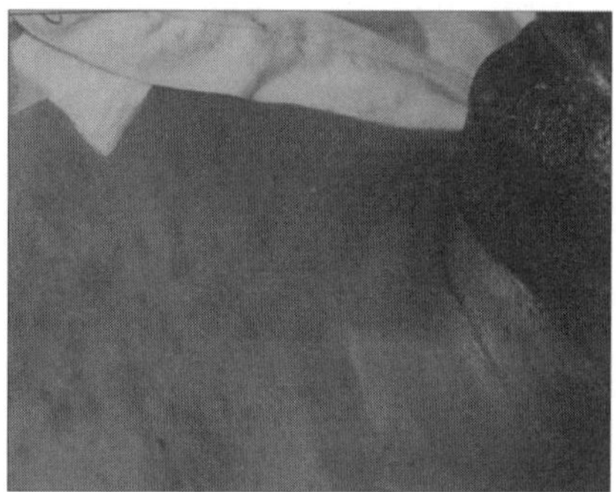

Fig. 11.9: Early erythema multiforme skin lesions will not be target-like and will be more prominent on the trunk and extremities

may resemble those of EM minor with a characteristic symmetrical distribution on the extremities. Nevertheless, the skin lesions may be atypical and characterized by bullae and affect a greater area (Fig. 11.9). If 10% or less of the body surface is affected then the disease fulfils the criteria for bullous EM (Bastuji-Garin, et al. 1993).

HSV-induced EM major is characterized by mucosal erosions plus typical or raised atypical targets and epidermal detachment involving less than 10% of the body surface and usually located on the extremities and/or the face.

Although EM minor and EM major have been described, the value of distinguishing clinically between them has been called into question. One large study of patients with recurrent EM showed that, in 90% of patients only one mucosal surface was affected in the primary attack but in subsequent episodes this proportion dropped to 61%, and in the other patients there were multiple mucosal sites affected (Farthing, et al. 1995). This indicates that patients who initially presented with apparent EM minor may present with EM major in subsequent attacks and that the minor and major forms of the disease are closely linked.

Stevens-Johnson Syndrome

Stevens-Johnson syndrome causes widespread lesions affecting the mouth, eyes, pharynx, larynx, esophagus, skin and genitals. It almost invariably involves the oral mucosa. A prodrome occurs in about 30% of cases, may begin within 1–3 weeks of starting a new drug and it lasts 1–2 weeks before the onset of the mucocutaneous manifestations, and presents with flu-like symptoms, sore throat, headache, arthralgias, myalgias, fever, bullous and other rashes, pneumonia, nephritis or myocarditis. Ocular changes, which resemble those of mucous membrane pemphigoid, dry eyes and symblepharon may result. Balanitis, urethritis and vulval ulcers may occur and it, may be followed by sicca syndrome, or even Sjögren's syndrome (de Roux Serratrice, et al. 2001).

Drug-induced SJS is characterized by mucosal erosions plus widespread distribution of flat atypical targets or purpuric macules and epithelial detachment involving less than 10% of body surface on the trunk, face and extremities.

Diagnosis

A diagnosis of EM can be difficult to readily establish, and there can be a need to differentiate from viral stomatitides, pemphigus, TEN and the subepithelial immune blistering disorders (pemphigoid and others) (Ayangco and Rogers, 2003).

There are no specific diagnostic tests for EM and the diagnosis is mainly clinical supported if necessary by biopsy. Biopsy of perilesional tissue, with histological and immunostaining examination are essential if a specific diagnosis is required. Biopsy shows intraepithelial edema and spongiosis early on, with satellite cell necrosis (individual eosinophilic necrotic keratinocytes surrounded by lymphocytes), vacuolar degeneration of the junctional zone and severe papillary edema with sub- or intra-epithelial vesiculation, and intense lymphocytic infiltration and immune deposits of fibrin and C3 at the basement membrane zone. There may be a perivascular lymphocytic infiltrate (CD4+ more than CD8+ T lymphocytes) with a few neutrophils and occasional eosinophils, and perivascular IgM, C3 and fibrin deposits. However, pathology can be variable and immunostaining is not specific for EM.

In EM major a complete blood count, urea and electrolytes, erythrocyte sedimentation rate (ESR), liver function tests, and cultures from blood, sputum and erosive areas should be taken. To identify an etiological agent it may be helpful to undertake serology for HSV or *M. pneumoniae*, or other micro-organisms.

Management

Spontaneous healing of EM can be slow—upto 2–3 weeks in minor and upto 6 weeks in major EM. Treatment is thus, indicated but controversial (Katz, et al. 1999).

No specific treatment is available but supportive care is important; a liquid diet and intravenous fluid therapy may be necessary. Early ophthalmological and dermatological consultation is needed for diagnosis and management. Precipitating factors, when identified, should be treated.

Antimicrobials may be indicated, acyclovir in HAEM or tetracycline in EM related to *M. pneumoniae.* A 5-day course of acyclovir at the first sign of lesions, or 400 mg qds for 6 months is useful for prophylaxis in HAEM. Continuous therapy of valacyclovir, 500 mg twice a day, has also been reported to be effective.

The use of corticosteroids is controversial. Minor EM may respond to topical corticosteroids, though systemic corticosteroids may be required and patients with major EM or SJS may need to be admitted for hospital care and should be treated with systemic corticosteroids (prednisolone 0.5–1.0 mg/kg)/day) tapered over 7–10 days) and/or azathioprine or other immunomodulatory drugs. 50% of SJS patients in one series required supplemental hydration or alimentation because of the severity of the oral cavity involvement (Stewart, et al. 1994).

Other treatments used, may include cyclophosphamide, dapsone, cyclosporine, azathioprine, levamisole and thalidomide (Schofield, et al. 1993; Conejo-Mir, et al. 2003). Plasmapheresis possibly has a place in the management of severe disease.

Oral antacids may be helpful for management of discrete oral ulcers. Electrolytes and nutritional support should be started as soon as possible. Oral hygiene should be improved with 0.2% aqueous chlorhexidine mouthwash.

TOXIC EPIDERMAL NECROLYSIS (LYELL'S SYNDROME)

Toxic epidermal necrolysis is a rare clinicopathologic entity, with a high mortality, characterized by extensive detachment of full thickness epithelium usually induced by drugs. The distinction of TEN from EM is unclear, but most cases are drug-induced and the lesions are extremely widespread. Drugs appear to trigger what appears to be an immunologically related reaction with sub and intraepithelial vesiculation. Recently, an increased number of cases in HIV/AIDS patients have been recorded.

Clinical Features

Toxic epidermal necrolysis presents with a cough, sore throat, burning eyes, malaise and low fever, followed after about 1–2 days by skin and mucous membrane lesions. The entire skin surface and oral mucosa may be involved, with upto 100% sloughing. Oral mucosae are involved in almost all cases. Gingival lesions are common and clinically are inflamed, with blister formation leading to painful widespread erosions.

Diagnosis of toxic epidermal necrolysis

Sheet-like loss of the epithelium and a positive Nikolsky sign are characteristic. Biopsy of perilesional tissue, with histological and immunostaining examination are essential to the diagnosis. Histopathologic examination is characteristic showing necrosis of the whole epithelium detached from the lamina propria.

Management of toxic epidermal necrolysis

Patients must be admitted to hospital as soon as possible to an intensive care unit for management.

DRUG-RELATED ERYTHEMA MULTIFORME

A wide range of drugs may give rise to EM (Table 11.1), and it may be impossible to clinically distinguish drug-induced EM from disease due to other causes (Roujeau, 1997; Ayangco and Rogers, 2003). Lesions typically affect the oral mucosa, the lips and bulbar conjunctivae. Initial bullae rupture to give rise to hemorrhagic pseudomembrane of the lips and widespread superficial oral ulceration. Other mucocutaneous surfaces less commonly affected include the nasopharyngeal, respiratory and genital mucosae.

Table 11.1: Drug-related EM (SJS and TEN)

Drugs most commonly implicated	*Drugs occasionally implicated*
Allopurinol	Busulfan
Barbiturates	Cephalosporins
Carbamazepine	Chlorpropamide
NSAIDs	Clindamycin
Penicillin	Codeine
Phenytoin	Ethambutol
Sulfonamides	Furosemide
	Gold
	Minoxidil
	Estrogens
	Phenothiazines
	Phenylbutazone
	Progestogens
	Protease inhibitors
	Rifampicin
	Tetracyclines
	Tolbutamide
	Vancomycin
	Verapamil

DRUG-RELATED TOXIC EPIDERMAL NECROLYSIS

Toxic epidermal necrolysis (Lyell syndrome) is clinically characterized by extensive mucocutaneous epidermolysis preceded by a macular or maculopapular exanthema and exanthema (Lyell, 1979; Rasmussen, et al. 1989). Intraorally, there is widespread painful blistering and ulceration of all mucosal mucosal surfaces. Toxic epidermolysis may be associated with antimicrobials (sulfonamides and thiacetazone), analgesics (phenazines), antiepileptics, allopurinol, chlormezanone, rifampicin, fluconazole and vancomycin (Ayangco and Rogers, 2003).

REFERENCE

1. Farthing P, Bagan JV, Scully C. Mucosal diseases series, Erythema multiforme. Oral Diseases 2005;11(4):261–7.

CHAPTER 12

Lupus Erythematosus

INTRODUCTION

Lupus erythematosus (LE) is a multisystem autoimmune disease associated with significant morbidity and mortality. Lupus erythematosus occurs most commonly in young women and ranges from mild cutaneous lesions and/or arthritis to renal failure or intense nervous, cardiac and hematological disturbances.[1]

The basic manifestations of LE occur in the connective tissue and blood vessels, but depending on the anatomical location and course of the disease, LE has been classified as:

- Systemic LE (SLE)
- Cutaneous LE (CLE).

Cutaneous lupus erythematosus includes variety of LE-specific skin lesions that are subdivided into 3 categories: Chronic CLE (CCLE), subacute CLE (SCLE) and acute CLE (ACLE) based on clinical morphology and histopathologic examination.

Patients with SLE frequently show cutaneous manifestations during the course of the disease. Moreover, 4 of the 11 criteria formulated by the American College of Rheumatology (ACR) classification for the diagnosis of SLE are cutaneous and oral. These criteria are malar rash, discoid rash, photosensitivity and oral ulcers.

Oral mucosal ulceration occurs in more than 40% of patients with SLE; however, reticular, red and white plaques have also been observed in patients with SLE. The majority of these lesions showed histopathological changes specific to SLE; however, histological and immunological patterns might be unspecific.

PATHOGENESIS

The characteristic disease findings in LE include inflammation, blood vessel changes such as vasculopathy, and immune-complex deposition. Generalized autoantibody production in SLE is a hallmark immunologic presentation, with antibodies directed to self-antigens of the nucleus, cytoplasm, cell surface, soluble IgG, and coagulation factors. Production of autoantibodies seems to mediate tissue injury by an immune complex mediated inflammatory response. Of particular importance to SLE are serum autoantibodies that are directed to a range of cell nucleus components such as DNA, RNA, nuclear proteins, and protein-nucleic acid complexes. These antinuclear antibodies (ANA) are found in 95% of SLE patients.

The specific antibodies to nuclear antigens are of particular importance to SLE. Antibodies to double-strand (ds) DNA (anti-ds DNA) and to nuclear antigen Smith (anti-Sm) target small nuclear ribonucleoprotein are unique to SLE, found in the sera of 40% and 30% of patients, respectively. ANA, anti-ds DNA, and anti-Sm are part of the classification criteria for SLE (Table 12.1). Other nuclear antigen antibodies found in SLE include anti-Ro, anti-La, anti-ribosomal P proteins (anti-P), and antiphospholipid. Although the clinical importance of specific nuclear antigen antibodies is not always clear, anti-ds DNA has been associated with glomerulonephritis. Other associations with clinical features of SLE include anti-P with psychosis and anti-Ro with congenital heart block and subacute cutaneous lupus. A recent study by Arbuckle demonstrated the relationship of ANA with disease progression.[2]

CLINICAL FEATURES

The presenting symptoms of SLE are often nonspecific constitutional signs such as fever, fatigue, and weight loss. Involvement of a variety of organs follows this initial presentation and can include mucocutaneous, renal, neurologic/psychiatric, cardiovascular and hematologic manifestations (Table 12.1). The disease course is characterized by disease flares, which may require immunosuppression for symptom management but which frequently decrease overtime, with periods of remission. Late mortality is more often related to cardiovascular disease. The 10-year survival has been estimated at 80%–90%, with early deaths often associated with infection secondary to immunosuppression.[2]

Table 12.1: Prevalence of disease manifestations and impact on dental care

Disease manifestation	*Prevalence (%)*	*Impact on dental care*
Mucocutaneous	80–90	Presence of acute oral lesions may cause discomfort. Consider SLE or DLE in differential diagnosis of oral lesions.
Renal disease	50–67	For patients requiring hemodialysis: Because of heparinization, provide dental treatment day after dialysis. Antibiotic prophylaxis may be requested by nephrologist to cover dialysis shunts, but concern for cardiac valvular damage is a better rationale for prophylaxis.

Contd...

Contd...

Disease manifestation	*Prevalence (%)*	*Impact on dental care*
Neuropsychiatric conditions	67	For patients with seizures, review history and type of seizures. Protect patient from harm if a seizure occurs during therapy. For patients with psychoses, ensure adequate medical management of condition.
Valvular damage	18–74	Use American Heart Association—It recommended antibiotic prophylaxis for confirmed cardiac valvular disease.
Severe coronary artherosclerosis	45	Evaluate blood pressure and coronary artery disease (CAD) symptoms (i.e. stable versus unstable angina). For advanced CAD, consider anxiolytics or defer treatment until patient is medically stable.
Infection	14–100	May have poor healing following invasive dental procedures. Evaluate closely postoperatively.
Anemia of chronic disease	80	Severe anemia may alter oxygen supply to organ systems. Evaluate laboratory values (i.e. complete blood cell count); may need to consider blood products with severe anemia (< 8 g/dL).
Leukopenia	50	Absolute neutrophil count (ANC) < 500 will predispose to infection. Evaluate laboratory values (i.e. complete blood cell count and differential); consider antibiotics after therapy with ANC < 500.
Thrombocy-topenia	25	Values $< 50 \times 10^9$/L may result in prolonged bleeding following invasive procedures. Evaluate laboratory values (i.e. complete blood cell count); consider platelet transfusion before invasive procedures with severe thrombocytopenia.
Antiphospho-lipid syndrome	14–20	Patients receiving warfarin may have increased bleeding following invasive procedures. Evaluate international normalized ratio (INR) before treatment. If INR < 3.5, no alteration in warfarin is usually necessary for invasive procedures. Use appropriate local measures for bleeding control. If INR > 3.5, discuss with physician appropriate measures to lower INR.

Contd...

Contd...

Disease manifestation	*Prevalence (%)*	*Impact on dental care*
Secondary Sjögren's syndrome	7.5–30	Increased incidence of caries and fungal infections. Consider use of parasympathomimetics (e.g. Pilocarpine or Cevimeline), fluoride gels, and antifungal agents with clinical evidence of a fungal infection.

MUCOCUTANEOUS DISEASE

Mucocutaneous involvement affects 80% to 90% of SLE patients. 4 of the 11 diagnostic criteria include mucocutaneous manifestations: Malar rash, discoid lesions, photosensitivity, and the presence of oral ulcerations (Box 12.1). Mucocutaneous manifestations of LE can be classified as chronic cutaneous lupus erythematosus (CCLE), subacute cutaneous lupus erythematosus (SCLE), and acute cutaneous lupus erythematosus (ACLE). The cutaneous and mucosal lesions of CCLE and SCLE can present alone or as part of the multisystem involvement of SLE. Patients with ACLE manifestations either have or will develop SLE.

Box 12.1: American College of Rheumatology criteria for systemic lupus erythematosus

1. Malar rash
2. Discoid lesions
3. Photosensitivity
4. Presence of oral ulcers
5. Nonerosive arthritis of two joints or more
6. Serositis
7. Renal disorder
8. Neurologic disorder (seizures or psychosis)
9. Hematologic disorder (hemolytic anemia, leukopenia, lymphopenia, or thrombocytopenia)
10. Immunologic disorder (anti-DNA, anti-Sm, or antiphospholipid antibodies)
11. Antinuclear antibody

Chronic Cutaneous Lupus Erythematosus

CCLE can have multiple mucocutaneous manifestations including discoid LE (DLE), hypertrophic DLE, lupus panniculitis, lupus tumidus, and chilblains LE.

Discoid Lupus Erythematosus

DLE is the most common form of CCLE and occurs in 15% to 30% of SLE patients; DLE also can exist without systemic disease. DLE lesions may occur at any age but occur most commonly during the 4th decade. Women are more commonly affected with DLE than men, by a 4.5:1 ratio.

Clinical Presentation

DLE lesions are characterized by erythematous plaques, frequently covered with a scale that tends to heal with scarring. The most common locations for DLE lesions are the face, scalp, ears, and neck, with the head and neck area affected in 80% of cases (Fig. 12.1),[2] DLE patients usually presents with no symptoms. Individuals will seek attention because of the development of dusky red localized skin plaques, 5–20 mm in diameter, on the face. These plaques will have a predilection for the hairline and sun exposed areas.

A butterfly malar rash develops in DLE, just as it does in SLE. The skin lesions are often referred to as "grass fire" lesions because, as they mature, they develop a broad atrophic white area with a perimeter of red resembling the pattern of a grass fire (Fig. 12.2). The scar within this white area will be devoid of hair follicles, leaving patchy bald areas in men's beards or a patchy alopecia on the scalp. In darker-skinned individuals, these lesions leave multiple depigmented regions. Some skin lesions will become scaly, resembling psoriasis.[3]

ORAL MANIFESTATIONS

The oral lesions usually manifest a central red atrophic area surrounded by white keratotic border lines, similar to their cutaneous counterpart. Most often they are present on the vermillion of the lip (Fig. 12.3) or on the buccal mucosa (Fig. 12.4). The labial lesions are prone to scale

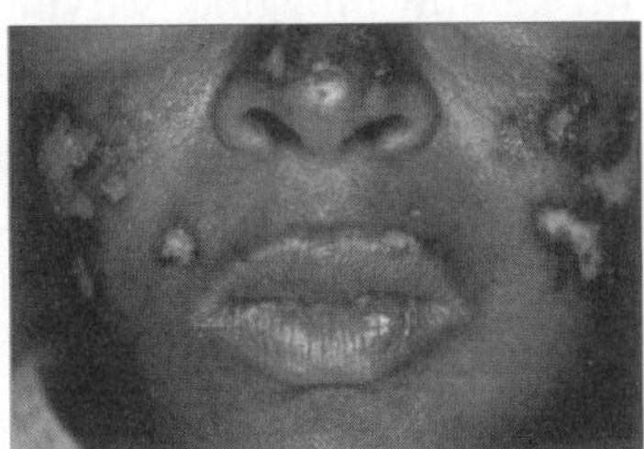

Fig. 12.1: Discoid lesions of the face characterized by pigment changes, scaling, and atrophy

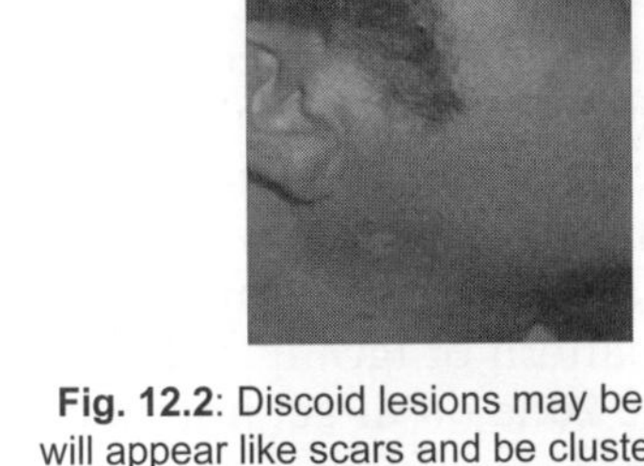

Fig. 12.2: Discoid lesions may be subtle but will appear like scars and be clustered around hair lines and in sun exposed areas

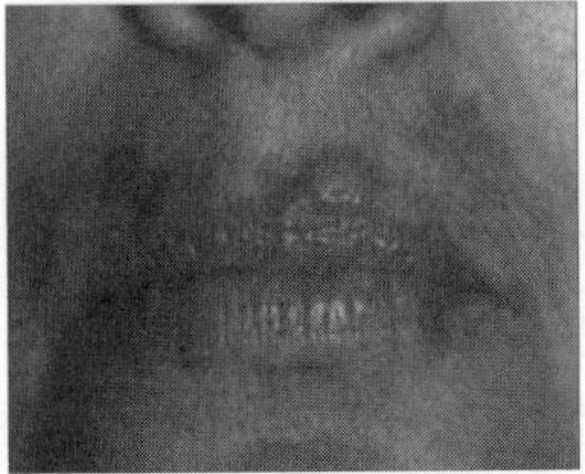

Fig. 12.3: Oral discoid lesions of the lip (red plaque-like areas are seen)

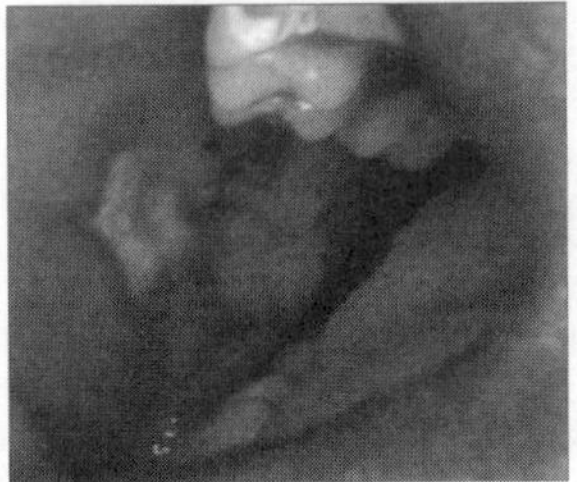

Fig. 12.4: Oral discoid lesions of the buccal mucosa (ulceration, plaque, and erythematous areas are seen)

formation, whereas those of the oral mucosa are not. Tongue lesions are associated with atrophy of the papillae. The hard palate and gingiva also may be involved. There may be increased tendency for individual with the discoid type to develop squamous cell carcinoma of the lower lip.

Differential Diagnosis

Cases that present with prominent skin ulcers, plaques, and perhaps oral lesions and a malar butterfly rash need to be distinguished from systemic lupus erythematosus. As an abbreviate screening test to rule out SLE, a battery of tests that include antinuclear antibodies (ANA), anti-double-stranded (native) DNA antibodies, and serum complement level is effective. All are negative or normal in DLE, whereas SLE yields at least one positive or abnormal finding. In particular, 95% of SLE patients will show hypocomplementemia because the systemic antigen-antibody complexes of that disease will consume; complement nearly to the point of depletion. The skin lesions also look like those of psoriasis, particularly if they are scaly and plaque like; skin tuberculosis (lupus vulgaris); sarcoidosis, or even an early lepromatous leprosy if similar multiple facial lesions are visible. Individual lesions may not be distinguishable from those of a sclerosing morphea type of basal cell carcinoma or seborrheic dermatitis.[3]

Histopathology

The microscopic changes associated with DLE include hyperkeratosis and/or hyperparakeratosis, sometimes with keratin plugging, varying areas of acanthosis and atrophy, hydropic degeneration of basal cells, and edema of the lamina propria and inflammatory infiltrates (Fig. 12.5). The inflammatory component is essentially lymphocytic and may be diffuse or perivascular in distribution. It often lies subjacent to the epithelium with cells migrating into the epithelium, known as an interface reaction, or it may be seen more deeply within the connective tissue in a perivascular arrangement. Most cases will demonstrate a granular pattern of IgG, IgM, IgA, C3, and fibrinogen in the basement membrane zone on direct immunofluorescence of involved mucosa of skin (Fig. 12.6).

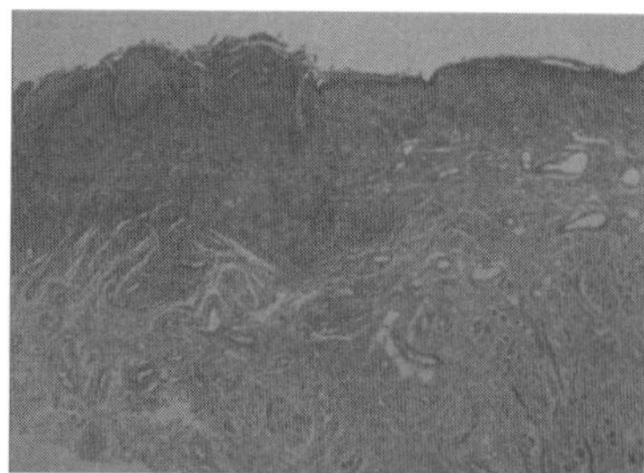

Fig. 12.5: Hyperplastic and atrophic areas with subepithelial lymphocytic infiltrate

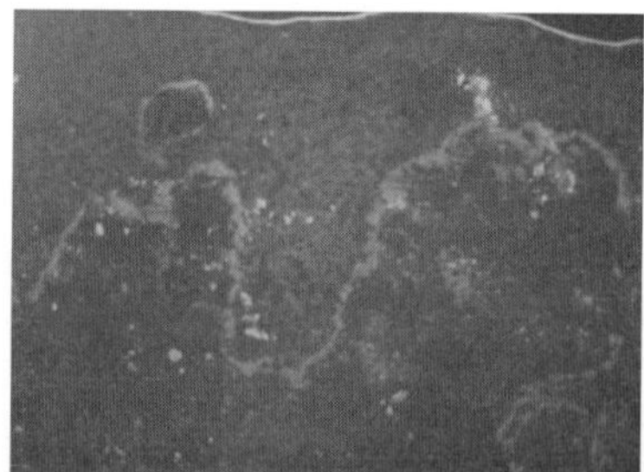

Fig. 12.6: Direct immunofluorescence showing a granular deposition of IgG in the basement membrane zone

The histologic features of DLE bear a close resemblance to those of lichen planus because both demonstrate an interface process with reactive epithelial changes. The feature that are more suggestive of lupus, and thus should be stressed, are the keratin plugs, the varied atrophy and acanthosis, connective tissue, edema, the deeper perivascular infiltrate and the less compact band of lymphocytes at the interface. In addition, immunoglobulins are identified in the basement membrane zone only in lupus.

Subacute cutaneous lupus erythematosus (SCLE)

SCLE is another subset of cutaneous lupus erythematosus, usually presenting in the 3rd to 4th decade of life. SCLE lesions appear in 7% to 27% of SLE patients and are characterized by erythematous, scaly papules or plaques that are more superficial than DLE lesions. SCLE lesions are more photosensitive, commonly occurring on sun exposed areas, (e.g. neck, shoulders, arms, chest, back). They primarily affect white women, and anti-Ro antibodies are a common presenting laboratory finding. The neck is most commonly affected (in 83% of SCLE patients), followed by the face (in 66% of SCLE patients).

Acute cutaneous lupus erythematosus (ACLE)

ACLE classically manifests as an erythematous/edematous rash that involves the malar eminences (butterfly rash), bridging the nose. Patients with ACLE lesions often meet the diagnostic criteria and ultimately develop SLE. The butterfly malar rash is seen in 30% to 60% of SLE patients. ACLE lesions are often triggered by sun exposure, and 33% to 67% of SLE patients have cutaneous or other systemic manifestations related to photosensitivity.

Systemic Lupus Erythematosus

Clinical presentation

Systemic lupus erythematosus is an autoimmune disorder in which antigen-antibody complexes become entrapped in the capillaries of most organs. These complexes initiate the complement cascade and inflammation. The clinical presentation, therefore, may show evidence of single-organ disease or wide spread multiorgan disease. It may also present in a mild episodic form or a rapidly progressive form leading to death, depending on the organs involved and the degree of autoimmune abnormality.

The classic presentation is a young woman of so-called childbearing age. 85% of patients are women, and indeed the peak incidence is between the ages of 20 and 40 years.

There is a higher incidence in blacks than in any other race, although it is not found in Africa. The most notorious feature of SLE is the malar butterfly rash (Fig. 12.7). However, the clinician should remember that other diseased such as DLE, pemphigus, and drug-induced conditions, can produce a similar rash and that the rash alone does not establish a diagnosis of SLE. In fact, the malar butterfly rash is only one of possible II clinical laboratory findings that may be present (Box. 12.1).

The American Rheumatism Association (ARA) requires that at least 4 of these 11 criteria be present, together with a positive serum ANA, before a definitive diagnosis of SLE can be made. Familiarity with these criteria helps the clinician know what to look for and which diagnostic tests to pursue.

In addition to the malar rash, which will usually spare the nasolabial crease there may be other skin lesions, known as a discoid rash (Fig. 12.8). These lesions are seen clustered around hairline areas and are exacerbated by exposure to sunlight (photosensitivity).

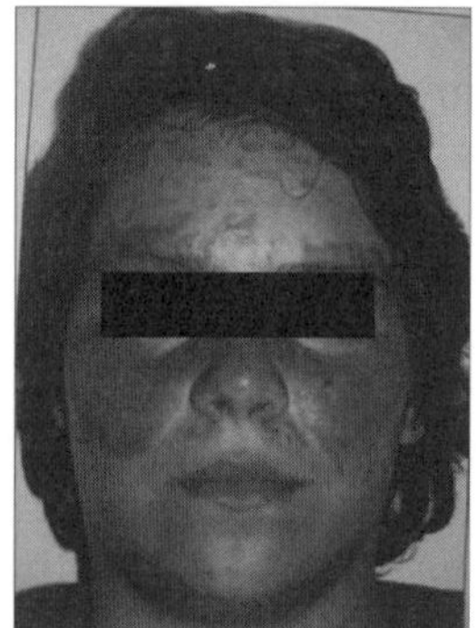

Fig. 12.7: SLE will often show the classic malar butterfly rash, which spares the nasolabial crease. Note the hairline cluster of other lesions around the eyebrow and forehead

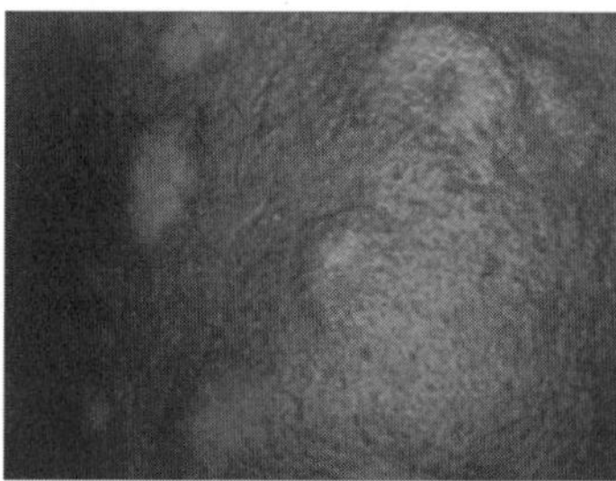

Fig. 12.8: The skin lesions of SLE will be like those of DLE and are called a discoid rash. In both they will form around hairlines and have the "grass fire" appearance

Mucosal lesions

Mucosal ulcerations in patients with SLE most commonly involve the mouth, nose, and anogenital region. These lesions may include DLE-type lesions or nonspecific LE ulcerations. Lesions in the oral cavity have been estimated to occur in 2% to 80% of SLE patients. The oral ulcers are red, shallow ulcers most commonly found on the palate (Fig. 12.9) and the marginal gingiva. At times, the oral lesions will take the form of a nonulcerated inflammatory area or a line of inflammation (Fig. 12.10). They may mimic a marginal gingivitis.

Joint symptoms (painful joints, mild swellings occur frequently in 90% of patients) and are often an early sign. This arthritis is not a deforming type of arthritis and will not show radiographic changes. Individuals with systemic lupus erythematosus also frequently exhibit Raynaud phenomenon. This phenomenon relates to color changes of the fingers in response to exposure to cold. It can be elicited by placing

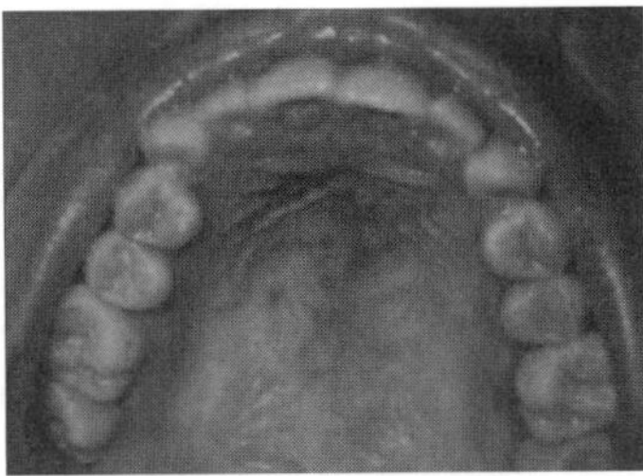

Fig. 12.9: Oral lesion of SLE seen on palate

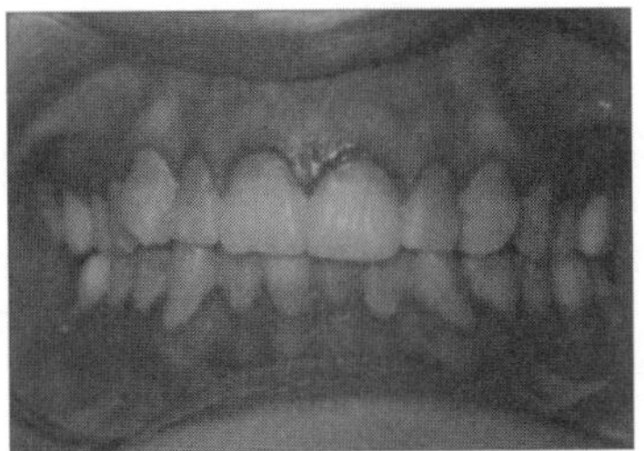

Fig. 12.10: Oral lesions of SLE involving marginal gingiva

the patient's hand in ice water, which will produce vasoconstrictions and vasodilatations, creating the so-called patriotic signs that are red, white, and/or blue changes in the skin color. Ocular manifestations include blurred vision, to transient blindness conjunctivitis, and photophobia. A slit-lamp or ophthalmoscopic examination may show fluffy cotton-wool spots, called cytoid bodies, on the retina.

Lung involvement will take the form of pleuritis with effusion, and there is also frequently a pneumonia and restrictive lung disease. The heart often develops pericarditis serositis and a verrucous nonbacterial endocarditis called Libman-Sacks endocarditis that is known to produce mitral valve regurgitations.

The renal disease takes the form of glomerulonephritis, mostly where glomerular thickening produces a wire loop nephritis also called lupus nephritis. Interstitial nephritis is also seen. The neurologic disease is often manifested as seizure activity and psychosis, particularly depression.[3]

Differential Diagnosis[3]

The most important differentiation to make when pursuing a suspected case of SLE is to distinguish from drug-induced lupus syndrome. In particular, methyldopa, hydralazine, chloropromazine, procainamide, isoniazid (INH), and quinidine have a strong association with the production of a lupus-like syndrome. To distinguish this clinically similar entity, the clinician must strictly adhere to the 11 ARA criteria and consider the following facts concerning a drug-induced lupus syndrome:

1. Males are affected equally
2. There are no neurologic or renal components
3. Antinative DNA antibodies are not present
4. The clinical picture improves if the suspicious drug is withdrawn.

Other diseases that may present with an initial picture similar to that of SLE include discoid lupus erythematosus, erythema multiforme, and rheumatoid arthritis.

Diagnostic Work-Up[3]

The physical examination and radiographic and laboratory studies are guided by the ARA criteria and are straightforward. There should be a routine urinalysis and a 24 hour urine collection specimen to assess for proteinuria and cellular casts indicative of glomerular damage. In addition, a routine chest auscultation, chest radiograph, and pulmonary function tests particularly assessing for pleural effusions, rev restrictive lung disease, and mitral valvular incompetence should be included.

The blood abnormalities in lupus are mainly cytopenia from marrow depression caused by immune effects. Therefore, a routine complete blood count should identify either anemia or leukopenia. Particularly lymphopenia, or thrombocytopenia. In addition, hypocomplementemia is commonly found in SLE (95% of cases) because the antigen-antibody complexes continually fix complement, thereby depleting their serum values. An ANA is required and is positive but is not specific for SLE. Other serum immunologic studies should include anti-DNA antibody, anti-Sm (Smith), which is a specific antiribonuclear proteins and a VDRL (Venereal Disease Research Laboratory) (the positive VDRL is often false positive in SLE). The antinative DNA antibody is reasonably specific for SLE, and when first introduced, was hoped to be a single diagnostic test for SLE, but its sensitivity is low. Only 30%–40% of SLE patients test positive for anti-DNA antibody.

HISTOPATHOLOGY[4]

The histologic changes of systemic lupus as observed in the oral mucosa do not differ appreciably from those in discoid lupus, and it has been observed that even the ulcerative lesions of SLE evolve from the same basic mechanism of destruction secondary to the interface reaction. In general, however, particularly in the early skin lesions of SLE, the changes may in degree. In these cases, connective tissue edema is more pronounced. As is hydropic degeneration of basal cells, and the inflammatory component and hyperkeratosis are diminished. Extravasation of erythrocytes is more pronounced and colloid bodies are more likely to be seen.

Deposits of fibrin are more prominent. This occurs within the connective tissue, causing thickening of collagen bundles, as well as within vessel walls and basement membrane zone (Fig. 12.11). These deposits are strongly PAS positive. Subcutaneous fat may also show involvement with mucoid degeneration and lymphocytic infiltrates. In

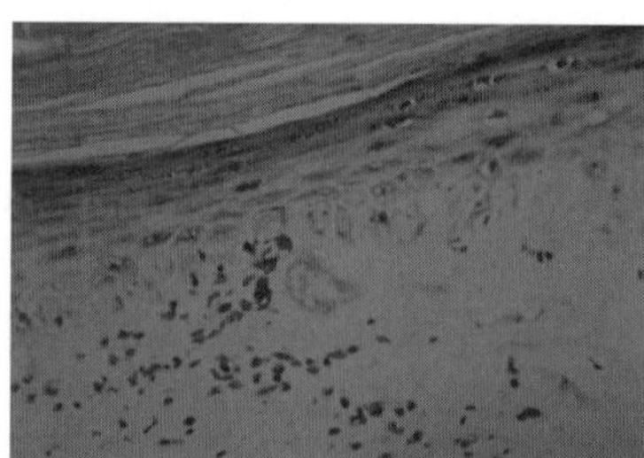

Fig. 12.11: SLE involving the skin, showing marked edema, scant inflammatory cells, extravasated erythrocytes, and some fibrin

virtually, all cases of SLE the granular deposits of immunoglobulin are seen on direct immunofluorescence (Fig. 12.6), a phenomenon that may also occur in cases of DLE.

Treatment of Mucocutaneous Disease

Guidelines from the American Academy of Dermatology for the management of cutaneous LE recommend: (Table 12.2)

1. Avoidance of sunlight with protective clothing or the use of at least UVB-15 protective sun blocks.
2. Topical or intralesional corticosteroids.
3. Systemic therapies including firstline medications of aminoquinoline antimalarial agents, dapsone, and prednisone. Approximately 50% to 80% of patients with cutaneous lupus respond to antimalarial agents.

For oral lesions, potent topical corticosteroids and antimycotic agents are often administered initially. Intralesional corticosteroids also may be considered. If there is no response with topical therapy, the use of antimalarial agents and more potent systemic therapies including steroids, Thalidomide, Clofazimine, and Methotrexate have been used.

Table 12.2: Topical therapy for oral lesions of lupus erythematosus

Topical steroid therapy[a]	*Directions for use*[b]
0.5% fluocinonide gel	Place on affected area(s) 2×/day for 2 weeks
0.5% clobetasol gel	Place on affected area(s) 2×/day for 2 weeks
Dexamethasone elixir (0.5 mg/5mL)	Swish and spit 10 mL 4×/day for 2 weeks
Triamcinolone acetonide 5 mg/mL	Intralesional injection
Topical antifungal therapy	
10 mg clotrimazole troches	Dissolve in mouth 5×/day for 10 days
Nystatin suspension (100,000 units/mL)	Swish and spit 5 mL 4×/day for 10 days
Chlorhexidine rinse (0.12%)	Swish and spit 10 mL 2×/day until lesions resolve

[a] Fungal infections are a side effect of topical steroids.
[b] If lesions do not respond appropriately to topical steroids in 2 weeks, consider systemic therapy such as antimalarials, steroids, thalidomide, clofazimine, and methotrexate.

Prognosis

The prognosis of patients with SLE improved in the 1980s. Currently, 10 year survival rates are of 85%. Most patients have a mild form of the disease requiring intermittent courses of prednisone. As the patient ages, the exacerbations become fewer and less intense, with longer disease-free remissions inbetween. After 5 years, the elevated erythrocyte sedimentation rate (ESR), ANA and anti-DNA antibody titters are reduced and may even be normal, because more SLE patients now survive for many years long-term corticosteroid complications, specially avascular necrosis of the hip and cataracts develop in most. A small number die from opportunistic infectious agents causing pneumonia.

If patient has virulent progressive course of SLE. It is evident from the onset. Those who survive first 4 years generally have long-term survival. The rapidly progressive form of SLE causes severe kidney damage heart damage, or lung damage leading to death mostly from renal failure or pneumonia.

Antiphospholipid Antibody Disease[3]

Antiphospholipid antibody disease may be part of the SLE picture exist as a separate primary antiphospholipid antibody syndrome. Antiphospholipid antibodies compose 32% of the autoantibodies found in SLE, and 3 different types are found. The first causes the biologic false-positive VDRL for syphilis and is found in 25% of SLE patients. The second is the lupus anticoagulant antibody, which, despite its name, causes both venous and arterial thrombosis, which in turn cause miscarriages. It is most commonly identified by an elevated partial thromboplastin time (PTT) and is found in 7% of SLE patients. The third type is an anticardiolipin antibody and has been associated with fetal death in pregnant women with SLE. It is found in 25% of SLE patients.

A primary antiphospholipid antibody syndrome unassociated with SLE also exists. Its main presentation is one of recurrent arterial and venous occlusions without any other features of SLE. Repeated venous or arterial occlusions in women and repeated unexplained miscarriages require a workup for SLE as well as antiphospholipid antibody determinations.

REFERENCES

1. Lopez-Labady J, Villarroel-Dorrego M. Oral manifestations of systemic and cutaneous lupus erythematosus in a Venezuelan population. J Oral Pathol Med 2007;36:524–7.
2. Brennan MT, Valerin MA, Napefias JJ, Lockhart PB. Oral manifestations of patients with lupus erythematosus. Dent Clin N Am 2005;49:127–41.
3. Marx RE, Stern D. Oral and Maxillofacial Pathology, Immune Based Diseases—Lupus Erythematosus. 2005;170–7.
4. Gorlin RJ, Goldman HM. Thoma's Oral Pathology, Mucocutaneous Disorders, 6th ed, 69–76.

CHAPTER 13

Epidermolysis Bullosa

INTRODUCTION

Epidermolysis bullosa (EB) forms a group of hereditary bullous disorders in which blisters form either spontaneously or they are triggered by trauma, having this denomination been suggested by Köebner in 1886.[1]

Epidermolysis bullosa (EB) encompasses a group of heterogeneous diseases of the skin and mucous membranes, which share the common feature of the formation of blisters and erosions in response to minor mechanical trauma. Most cases of EB are inherited. A comprehensive classification based on clinical presentation, genetic pattern of inheritance and electron microscopic features was proposed in 1991 by the subcommittee of the National EB Registry. EB is classified into 3 groups by the level at which the separation occurs:[2]

- EB simplex (EBS; intraepidermal skin separation)
- Junctional EB (JEB; skin separation in lamina lucida)
- Dystrophic EB (DEB; sublamina densa separation).

Researchers recently have proposed a new category termed hemidesmosomal EB (HEB), which exhibits splitting at either the intracellular or extracellular domains of the hemidesmosome. EBS is usually associated with little or no extracutaneous involvement, while the more severe hemidesmosomal, junctional, and dystrophic forms of EB may produce significant multiorgan system involvement, involving the mucosal surface of the mouth, esophagus, stomach, intestines, upper airway, bladder, and the genitals.[3]

PATHOGENESIS[1]

Basal keratinocytes connect to the dermis through the basal membrane area (dermoepidermical junction), as evidenced by SPA (Schiff's periodic acid) under optic microscopy as a fine, homogenous linear region. Under electron microscopy, 2 regions are observed: lamina lucida, which is electron-sparse, below basal keratinocytes, and another, lamina densa or basalis, above the dermal area that binds to the upper portion of the latter by anchoring fibrils, which are electron dense filaments.[1]

Under optical microscopy, EBs present with blisters in the subepidermal region and, observing this region under electron microscopy, over 16 subtypes were observed and gathered in 3 main groups (Fig. 13.1).[1,3]

1. **Epidermolysis bullosa simplex**—There is an intraepidermal cleavage at the lower portion, owing to cytolytic alterations of basal keratinocytes with defects in cytokeratines 5 (KRT5 gene) and 14 (KRT14 gene).[4] Subtypes: Köebner, Weber-Cockaine, Dowling-Meara and Ogna's variant.
2. **Epidermolysis bullosa junctionalis**—Cleavage occurs at lamina lucida or at the central region of the basal membrane area, the ceiling being represented by epidermis and the floor by lamina densa. It is owed to alterations in laminin-5 (LAMA3, LAMB3, LAMC2 genes), integrin-a6b4 (ITGA6 and ITGB4 genes) and transmembrane collagen XVII (COL17A1 gene), being the same as bullous pemphigoid antigen.[4] Subtypes: Herlitz, non-Herlitz benign generalized atrophic.
3. **Epidermolysis bullosa dystrophica**—Cleavage ocurrs at sublamina densa. Epidermis and lamina lucida represent the ceiling of the blister and dermis represents the floor. Alteration is exclusively in COL7A1 gene.[4] Subtypes: Cockaine-Touraine, Pasini, Hallopeau-Siemens and the recessive mitis dystrophic form.

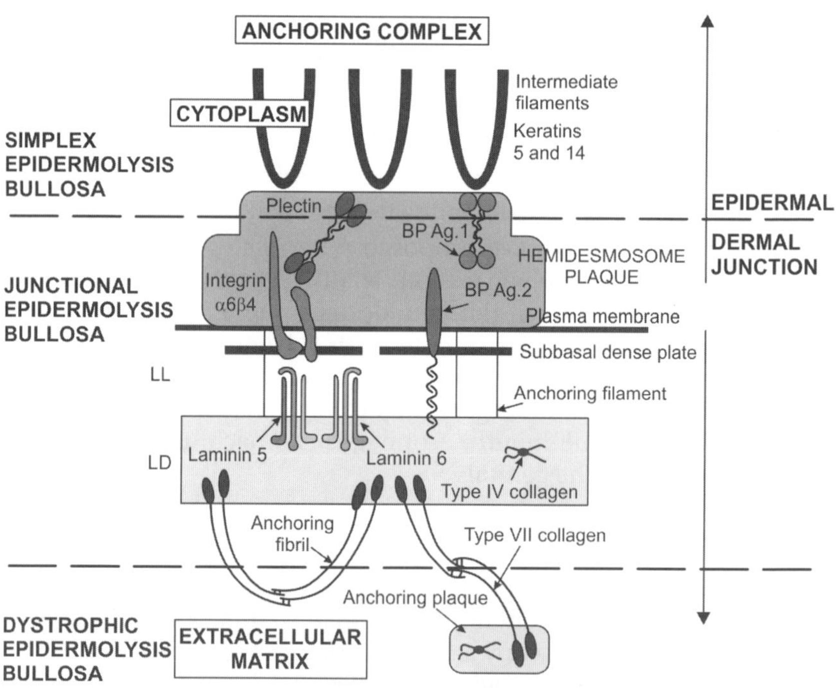

Fig. 13.1: Principal components and their relative localization in the anchoring complex of the epidermal-dermal junction, and their correspondence to major types of epidermolysis bullosa. LL—Lamina lucida, LD—Lamina densa

Acquired epidermolysis bullosa is an autoantibody-mediated disease, in which these antibodies deposit on lamina and sublamina densa, emerge in adulthood, with formation of blisters in areas submitted to trauma, which heal with atrophic scars and milium. In this type of EB there is no mutation, however, immunogenetic studies have demonstrated a connection with HLA DR2.

In EB, both dominant and recessive inheritance patterns are found, upto this date with no association with histocompatibility antigens (HLA).

EPIDERMOLYSIS BULLOSA SIMPLEX

Clinical Features

The generalized form of epidermolysis bullosa simplex is inherited as an autosomal dominant characteristic, manifest itself at birth or shortly thereafter and is characterized by the formation of vesicles and bullae, chiefly on the hands and feet at sites of friction or trauma. The knees, elbows and trunk are only occasionally affected. When the blisters heal, usually within 2–10 days, it is an important feature that there is no resultant scarring or permanent pigmentation. The disease appears to improve at puberty and prognosis is good for a normal lifespan.[4]

The localized form of the disease (Weber-Cockayne syndrome), which is also familial may occur early in childhood or later in life and is commonly recurrent. The bullae only develop on the hands and feet, are related to frictional trauma and tend to exacerbate in hot weather. There is no scarring upon healing (Fig. 13.2).

Oral Manifestations

Bullae of the oral cavity have been reported in occasional cases of generalized epidermolysis bullosa simplex, but it is doubtful that they actually occur. In addition, the teeth are not affected (Fig. 13.3).

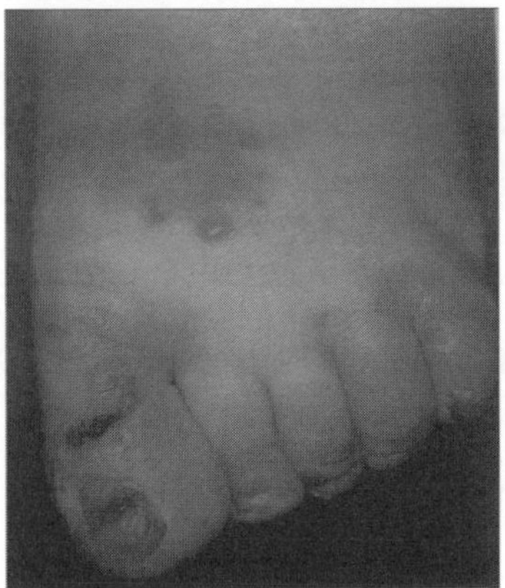

Fig. 13.2: EB simplex with small superficial bullae that heal without scarring

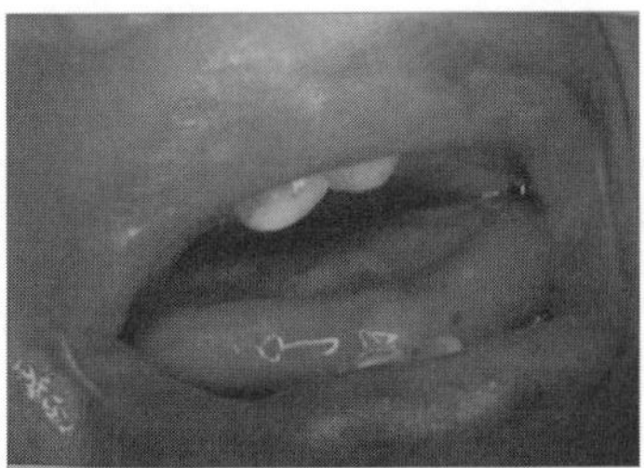

Fig. 13.3: EB simplex with muscular dystrophy frequently forms bullae of the oral mucosa

Histologic Features

In the generalized form of epidermolysis bullosa simplex, the vesicles and bullae develop as a result of destruction of basal and suprabasal cells so that some nuclei may persist on the floor of the blister, according to Lowe. The individual cells become edematous and show dissolution of organelles and tonofibrils with displacement of the nucleus to the upper end of the cell. The PAS (periodic acid-Schiff) positive basement membrane remains on the dermal side of the separation. The elastic, pre-elastic and oxytalan fibers in the connective tissue are normal.

In the localized form of the disease, the bullae are intra-epidermal and suprabasal in location.

JUNCTIONAL EPIDERMOLYSIS BULLOSA

It was earlier suggested by some workers that the junctional or lethal type is simply an extremely severe form of the dystrophic recessive form which is incompatible with prolonged survival. However, recent studies have proven that the two are distinctly different disorders.[4]

Clinical Features

Three criteria have been established for the diagnosis of this form of the disease. These are:

- Onset at birth
- Absence of scarring, milia or pigmentation
- Death within 3 months of age.

The bullae are similar to those seen in the dystrophic recessive type except that they commonly develop spontaneously, and sheets of skin may actually be shed.

Oral Manifestations

Oral bullae are frequently very extensive, and because of their extreme fragility, produce serious feeding problems. Similar lesions also occur in the upper respiratory tract, the bronchioles and the esophagus.

Severe disturbances in enamel and dentin formation of the deciduous teeth also occur but this is of only academic interest. These have been described by Gardner and Hudson in significant detail.

Histologic Features

The microscopic changes, including the location of the bullous cleavage, appear similar and probably identical to those occurring in the dystrophic recessive disease (Fig. 13.4).

EPIDERMOLYSIS BULLOSA DYSTROPHIC, DOMINANT

Clinical Features

This form of the disease may have its onset in infancy or it may be delayed until puberty. The blisters commonly develop on the ankles, knees, elbows, feet and head; healing results in scarring which is sometimes keloidal in type. In the majority of cases, the nails are thick and dystrophic, and milia are commonly present. However, the eye is never involved. Palmar-plantar keratoderma with hyperhydrosis also may occur as well as ichthyosis and sometimes hypertrichosis (Fig. 13.5).

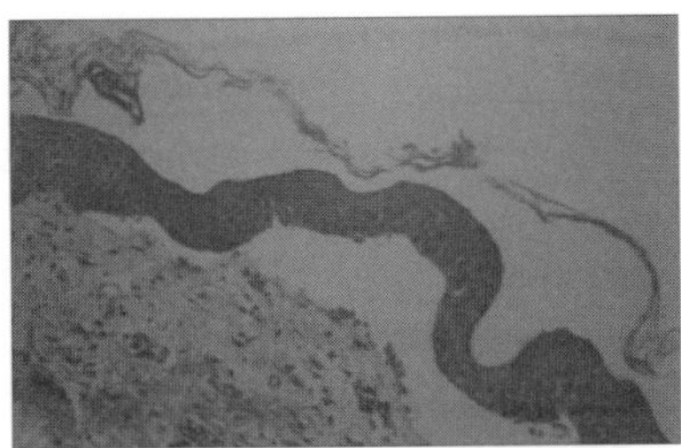

Fig. 13.4: Complete separation of the epithelium from the connective tissue (Junctional epidermolysis bullosa)

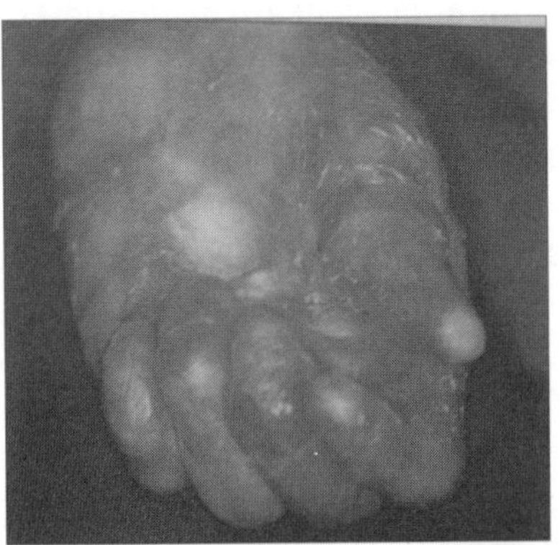

Fig. 13.5: Dominant dystrophic EB/ hypertrophic form with dystrophic nails, prominent scarring and thick skin pads

Oral Manifestations

Bullae of the oral cavity have been described as occurring in about 20% of cases of this type, and Andreasen has described oral milia. The teeth are unaffected.

Histologic Features

The bullae in this form of the disease develop as a result of separation through the very thin, irregular PAS-positive basement membrane which becomes divided. The basal layer appears normal although flattened on the roof of the blister. The underlying connective tissue shows an absence of elastic and oxytalan fibers.

EPIDERMOLYSIS BULLOSA DYSTROPHIC, RECESSIVE

Clinical Features

This type of EB is the best known and classic form of the disease. It has its onset at birth or very shortly, thereafter, and is characterized by the formation of bullae spontaneously or at sites of trauma, friction or pressure. The typical sites of involvement are the feet, buttocks, scapulae, elbows, fingers and occiput. The bullae contain a tinged fluid. When these bullae rupture or are peeled off under trauma or pressure, they leave a raw, painful surface. These patients frequently have a positive Nikolsky's sign. The bullae heal by scar, milia and pigmentation. This scarring may result in a functional club-like fist. The hair may be sparse while the nails are usually dystrophic or absent.

Oral Manifestations

Oral bullae are common in this form of the disease. They may be preceded by the appearance of white spots or patches on the oral mucous membrane or the development of localized areas of inflammation. The bullae may be initiated by nursing or by any simple dental operative procedure in the oral cavity. Unless great caution is used, large areas of mucous membrane may be inadvertently denuded. These bullae are painful, specially when they rupture or when the epithelium desquamates. Scar formation often results in obliteration of sulci and restriction of the tongue. Hoarseness and dysphagia may occur, as a result of bullae of the larynx and pharynx. Esophageal involvement may produce serious stricture.

Dental defects have also been described, consisting of rudimentary teeth, congenitally absent teeth, hypoplastic teeth and crowns denuded of enamel. These have been discussed in detail by Arwill and his associates.

Histologic Features

The separation and bulla formation here occur immediately beneath the poorly defined PAS-positive basement membrane which remains attached to the roof of the blister. Fragments of the basement membrane may adhere to the dermis, however. The basal layer of cells is normal. The pre-elastic and oxytalan fibers in the connective tissue are also increased but appear fragmented, according to Lowe.

Treatment

This group of diseases cannot be cured so that therapy is chiefly symptomatic. The simplex form of the disease requires little treatment; the lethal form will terminate fatally in most cases regardless of management. In the dystrophic forms prevention of trauma may reduce the incidence of bulla formation, but this is almost impossible to achieve. Antibiotics are useful in controlling secondary infection and cortisteroids have sometimes been found effective. EB is a lifelong disease. Some subtypes, specially the milder EB forms, improve with age.

REFERENCES

1. Gürtler Thaiz Gava Rigoni, Diniz Lucia Martins, João Basilio de Souza Filho. Recessive dystrophic epidermolysis bullosa mitis—Case report; An Bras Dermatol 2005;80(5):503–8.
2. Kao CH, Chen SJ. Junctional epidermolysis bullosa. J Chin Med Assoc 2006;69(10):503–6.

3. Hon Kle, Choi Pcl, Burd A, Luk NM. Epidermolysis bullosa dystrophica in a Chinese Neonate. HK J Paediatr (new series) 2007;12:137–43.
4. Shafer-Hine. Levy Textbook of Oral Pathology, 5th ed.

CHAPTER 14

Darier's Disease

(**Synonyms**: Keratosis follicularis, dyskeratosis follicularis)

INTRODUCTION

Darier is a rare keratinization disorder. It is an autosomal dominant genodermatosis with high penetrance and variable expressivity. Its manifestations appear in childhood and adolescence. The clinical signs are represented by several hyperkeratotic papules primarily affecting seborrheic areas on the head, neck, thorax, hand palms and foot soles, and less frequently the oral mucosa.[1]

Darier disease was initially described by Prince Marrow in 1886 and simultaneously by Darier and White in 1889, independently. The first report of mucosal manifestations was described by Reenstierna in 1917.[1]

The prevalence of this disorder in the population is 1:100,000, most often affecting males. The oral mucosa is affected in 50% of cases, in these cases, lesions are usually asymptomatic and discovered during routine dental examination.[1]

PATHOGENESIS

The condition is inherited as an autosomal dominant trait having high degree of penetrance and variable expressivity. The primary features are abnormal cell-cell adhesion and aberrant epidermal keratinization. Electron microscopy reveals loss of desmosome-keratin intermediate filament attachment, and perinuclear aggregates of keratin intermediate filaments.

These observations suggest that the molecules responsible for cell-cell adhesion, such as desmosomal catherins, desmosomal plaque proteins, or intermediate filament proteins, may be involved in the disease process. However, recently, mutations in the gene ATP2A2 gene (located at 12q23-q24.1) were fond in patients with Darier's disease.[2] This gene encodes the sarco/endoplasmic reticulum calcium pumping ATPase (SERCA2), which is highly expressed in keratinocytes. The magnesium dependent enzyme catalyzes the hydrolysis of ATP coupled with the transport of the calcium. It transports calcium ions from the cytosol into the sarcoplasmic/endoplasmic reticulum and has a central role in intracellular calcium signaling.

The gene encodes for 2 isoforms generated by alternative splicing: class 1/ATP2A2a and class 2/ATP2A2b that differ in their carboxy termini and have distinct tissue-expression patterns.[6] The first is located primarily in heart and slow-twitch skeletal muscle, whereas SERCA2b is present in smooth muscle and nonmuscle tissues. In adult skin sections only the longer isoform, SERCA2b is detected.[3] For pathomechanism of Darier's disease see Flowchart 14.1.[4]

Function of SERCA[4]

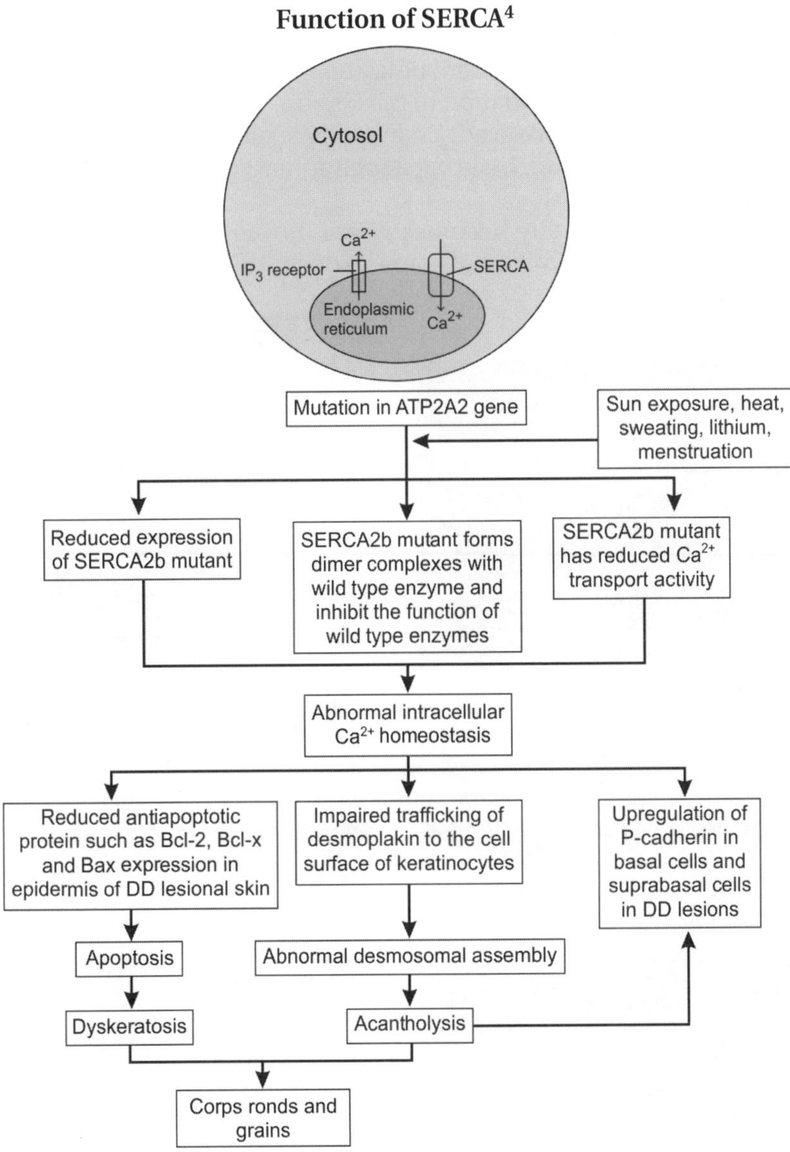

Flowchart 14.1: Pathomechanism of Darier's disease

CLINICAL FEATURES

Keratosis follicularis is usually manifested during childhood or adolescence and has an equal gender distribution. The cutaneous lesions appear as small, firm papules, which are red when they first appear, but characteristically become grayish brown or even purple, ulcerate and crust over. Specially in the skin folds, the lesions tend to coalesce and produce verrucous or vegetating macerated, foul smelling masses. They are generally distributed about the forehead, scalp, neck and over the shoulders, but often spread to the limbs, chest and genitalia (Figs 14.1 to 14.3). Palmar and plantar keratotic thickening (Figs 14.4 and 14.5) may be so severe as to interfere with function, and is associated with foul odor as a result of bacterial degradation of the keratin. In severe cases, all the intertriginous areas are involved. Characteristic nail changes are also seen consisting of splintering, fissuring, longitudinal streaking (Fig. 14.6) and subungual keratosis.[2]

The process generally becomes worse during the summer months, either because of sensitivity of some patients to ultraviolet light or be-

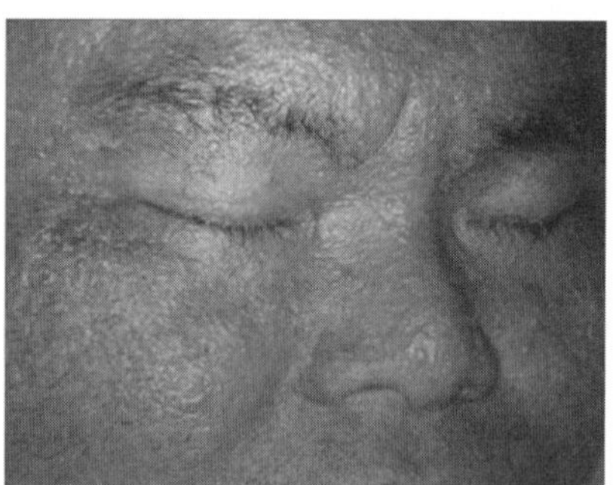

Fig. 14.1: Hyperkeratotic papules coalesce to form extensive flesh-colored plaques over face

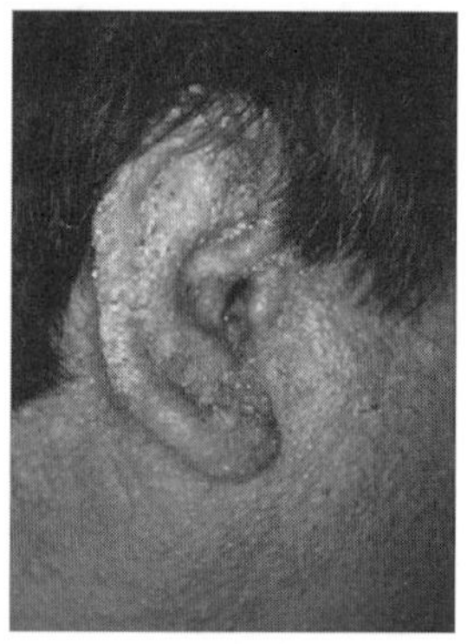

Fig. 14.2: Numerous hyperkeratotic papules with overlying greasy scaling over ears and periauricular region

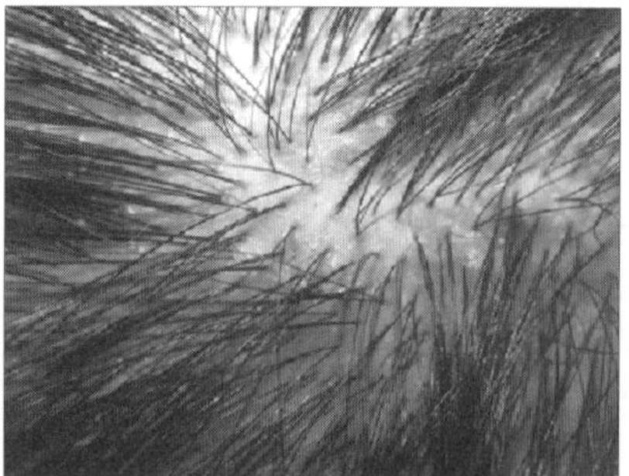

Fig. 14.3: Greasy hyperkeratotic papules over the scalp

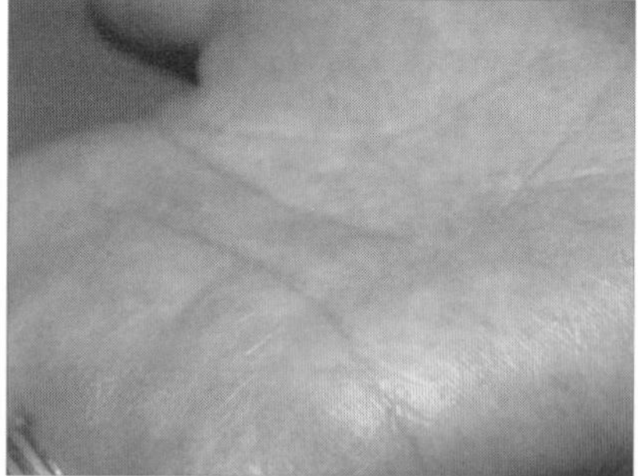

Fig. 14.4: Palmar pits and punctate keratosis over right hand

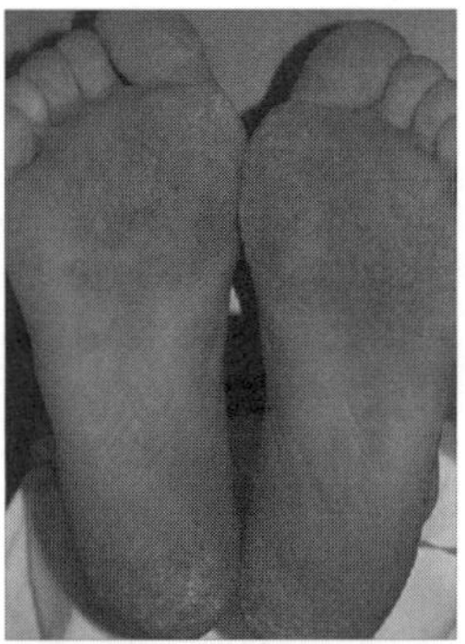

Fig. 14.5: Punctate keratosis and pitting over soles

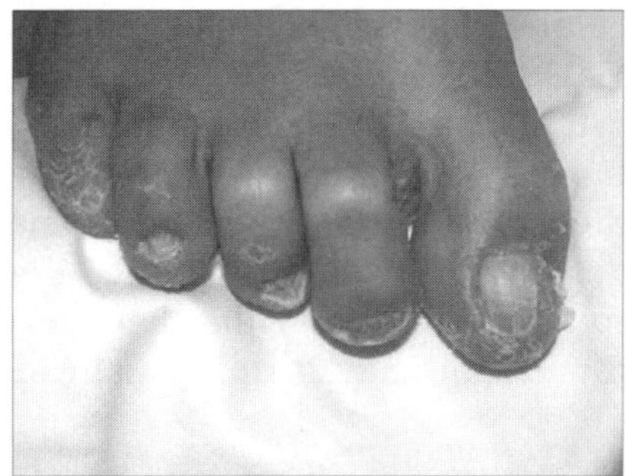

Fig. 14.6: Nail ridging and splitting of toe nails

cause increased heat results in sweating, which induces more epithelial clefting.[5]

Oral Manifestations

The oral lesions are typically asymptomatic and are discovered on routine examination. The frequency of occurrence of oral lesions ranges from 15%–50%. They consist of multiple, normal-colored or white flat topped papules that, if numerous enough to be confluent, results in a cobblestone mucosal appearance. These lesions affect the hard palate (Fig. 14.7) and alveolar mucosa primarily, although the buccal mucosa or tongue may be occasionally involved. If the palatal lesions are prominent, the condition may resemble inflammatory papillary hyperplasia or nicotine stomatitis. Some patients with this condition also experience recurrent obstructive parotid swelling secondary to duct abnormalities.[5]

Histologic Features

The histologic picture of Darier disease includes hyperkeratosis/hyperparakeratosis and acanthosis, sometimes with papillomatosis. One of the characteristic features, however, is suprabasal acantholysis, which results in the formation of suprabasilar separations or lacunae. At the lacunar base, villus projections may develop into the space, and the basal cells can proliferate as narrow cords into the connective tissue. In addition to these horizontal separations, vertical clefts may be seen extending into the surface of the epithelium. The underlying connective tissue usually will show varying amounts of chronic inflammation (Fig. 14.8).

Two types of benign dyskeratotic cells can be seen in Darier disease. Corps ronds (i.e. round bodies) are rounded epithelial cells with a homogeneous, eosinophilic material. The periphery of the cells consists of basophilic dyskeratotic material. These cells are usually seen in the upper layers of epithelium. Grains are epithelial cells with elongated nuclei and basophilic or eosinophilic cytoplasm that are seen in the keratin layers or within lacunae (Figs 14.9 and 14.10).

Ultrastructurally, the corps ronds show extensive vacuolation of the cytoplasm with bundles of tonofilaments at the periphery. Grains show nuclear remnants, compression of vacuoles, and bundles of tonofilaments throughout the cytoplasm. The tonofilaments separate from the desmosomes and proliferate, creating the dyskeratotic process. Corps ronds and grains, while characteristic of the disease, are not pathognomonic, and they are not usually present in oral mucosal lesions.[6]

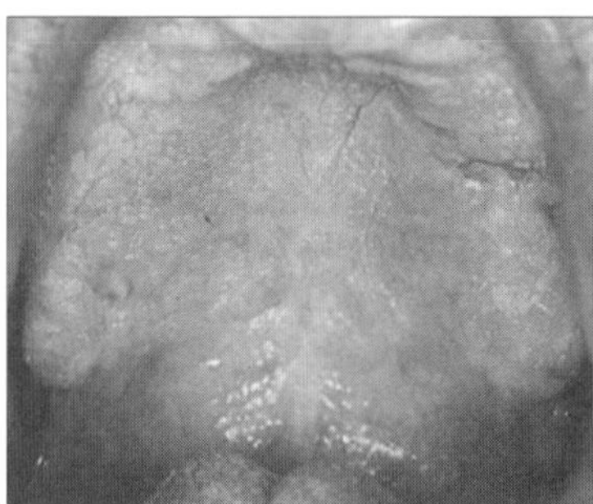

Fig. 14.7: Mucosal alterations on the hard palate represented by the presence of multiple coalesced papules with rugose texture

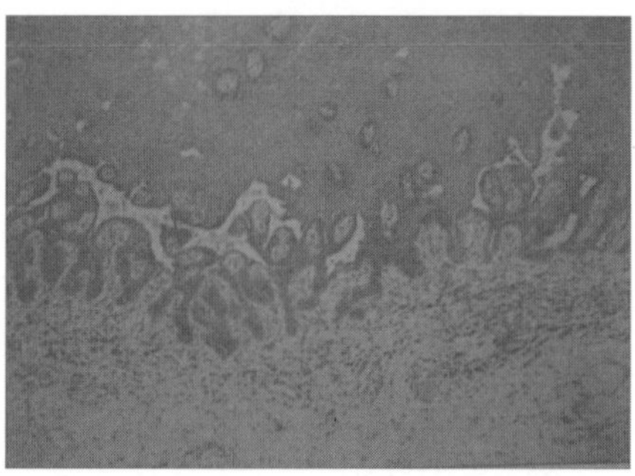

Fig. 14.8: Small suprabasilar separations called lacunae, as well as some vertical clefts. A chronic inflammatory infiltrate is apparent

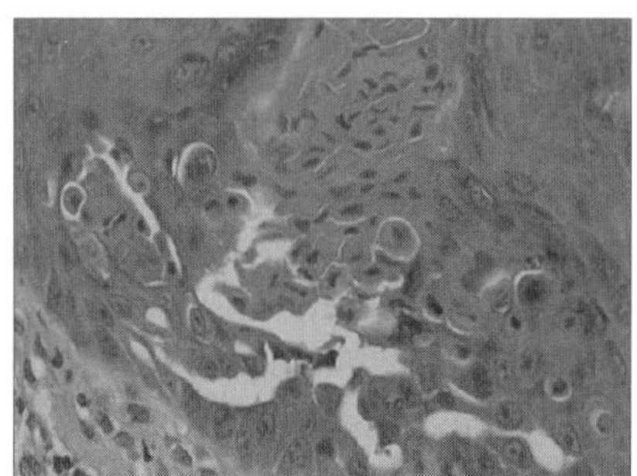

Fig. 14.9: Close up view shows the acantholysis, corps ronds and grains in detail

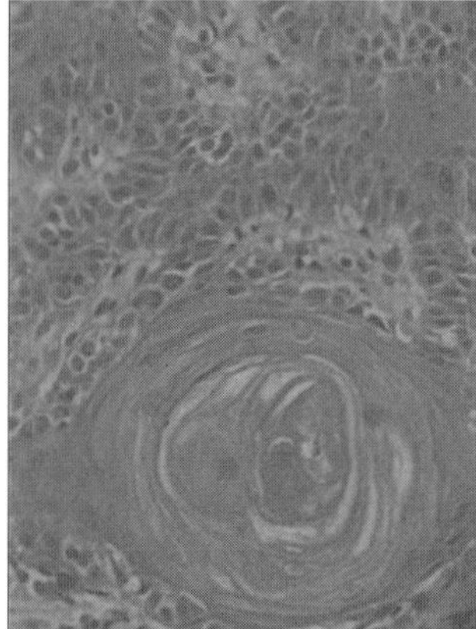

Fig. 14.10: Dyskeratotic cells observed as corps ronds

DIAGNOSIS

Regardless of the clinical severity and treatment option, the patient should receive genetic counseling with information on the inherited condition and risk of transmission to the offspring. Most often, dental doctors diagnose the oral manifestations in routine examinations before medical doctors, since lesions are asymptomatic. Biopsy is fundamental to allow final diagnosis; based on this result, the patient should be referred to dermatological examination.

Differential Diagnosis

The distinctive odor and greasy brown to black keratotic plugs are somewhat pathognomonic. However, less advanced cases will bear a clinical resemblance to the two pachyonychia congenita syndromes, *Jodassohn-Lewandowsky* syndrome and *Jackson-Lawler* syndrome, both of which have a component of hyperkeratosis particularly involving palms, soles and nail beds. However, the degree of hyperkeratosis never becomes as prominent as in Darier disease, and these 2 syndromes begin or are noticed just after birth. Similarly, the thickened and darkly hyperpigmented skin associated with palmar and plantar hyperkeratosis in the malignant form of *acanthosis nigricans* may resemble Darier disease; however, the axillary, genital and neck distribution in *acanthosis nigricans* as well as the lack of odor should distinguish the two. *Papillon-Lefevre* syndrome is also associated at times with dramatic palmar and plantar keratosis but lacks skin lesions elsewhere and is associated with alveolar bone loss and tooth mobility.[6]

TREATMENT

The systemic treatment of the Darier disease is symptomatic. The lesions relapse because of the hereditary etiopathogenesis, specially in patients with the severe and generalized form of the disease, who are usually treated with systemic and topical retinoids and in whom oral lesions still persist.[1]

Thus, therapies mentioned in the literature have a cosmetic goal, aiming at improving the patient's quality of life with regard to esthetics and specially hygiene, which may be improved in the oral cavity by utilization of nonalcoholic mouthrinses, since the coalescence of papules in skin or mucosa leads to accumulation of organic products (keratin degraded by bacteria), which causes a bad odor and favors the accumulation of microorganisms, producing secondary infection. Some authors mention that these complications are worsened by heat.[1]

Several treatments have been presented in the literature, such as utilization of topical retinoids, steroids and antibiotics; however, they provide limited benefits. Medical therapy includes utilization of systemic retinoids due to their efficacy; however, they should be carefully described by the medical doctor. More radical treatments have been reported, including surgical excision, abrasion, application of carbon dioxide and laser. Photodynamic therapy has been also considered; however, authors believe that it should not replace systemic retinoids in patients requiring systemic treatment. Utilization of topical 1% vitamin A acid is advocated in dyskeratoses, yet favorable outcomes have not been reported.[1]

REFERENCES

1. Cardoso CL, Freitas P, Taveira LA de A, Consolaro A. Darier disease: Case report with oral manifestations. Med Oral Patol Oral Cir Bucal 2006;11:E404–6.
2. Shafer, Hine, Levy Textbook of Oral Pathology, 5th ed.
3. Nives Peina-laus, Vinja Milavec-Pureti. Clinical case of acral hemorrhagic Darier's disease is not caused by mutations in exon 15 of the ATP2A2 Gene; Coll Antropol 27 (2003) 1:125–33 UDC 616.5–056.7:575.224.2; Original scientific paper.
4. Hoi CY. Darier's disease (keratosis follicularis) a local survey, study of life impact, mutation analysis of the ATP2A2 gene and review dissertation submitted in part fulfillment for Higher Physician Training in Specialty of Dermatology & Venereology, Hong Kong College of Physicians, 2004.
5. Neville, Damm, Allen, Bouquot. Oral and Maxillofacial Pathology, 2nd ed. Dermatologic diseases.
6. Marx. Oral and Maxillofacial Pathology.

CHAPTER

15

Dyskeratosis Congenita

(**Synonyms**: Zinsser-Engman-Cole syndrome, Hoyeraal-Hreidarsson syndrome)

INTRODUCTION

Dyskeratosis congenita (DC) is a rare syndrome, with approximately 180 individuals reported in the literature.[2] It was first described by Zinsser in 1906. Later Engman and Cole, et al. reported other cases in detail and hence it is also known as Cole-Engman syndrome or Zinsser-Cole-Engman syndrome. DC occurs mostly in males and manifests between 5 to 12 years. Classic triad of skin pigmentation, nail dystrophy and oral leukoplakia occur in complete expression of this syndrome. DC is a fatal condition in which majority of the patients develop aplastic anemia and malignant transformation occur in the keratotic white patches which is of considerable interest to a dentist.[1]

PATHOGENESIS

DC is a fatal condition with multisystem manifestations. There are X-linked, autosomal dominant and autosomal recessive forms of DC. It mainly occurs in the males, inherited as X-linked recessive disorder with male:female predilection of 13:1. Occurrence in extremely low percentage of the females suggests that there are subsets inherited in an autosomal dominant fashion. Autosomal dominant form of dyskeratosis congenita is associated with mutations in the RNA component of telomerase, hTERC, while X-linked dyskeratosis congenita is due to mutations in the gene encoding dyskerin, a protein implicated in both telomerase function and RNA processing. In DC multiple organ systems are affected due to pleiotropic mutation in the gene.[1]

CLINICAL FEATURES

Dyskeratotic congenita usually becomes evident during first 10 years of life.

Dermatologic Manifestations

It occurs in form of reticular hyperpigmentation of skin. These pigmented areas are associated with atrophy of epidermis, capillary hyperplasia and melanin pigment deposited near the blood vessels (Fig. 15.1). Dystrophy of nails is associated with the onset of skin pigmentation. Nail abnormalities can result in longitudinal splitting and furrowing. Nails are brittle or completely lost (Figs 15.2 and 15.3).

In DC eye involvement can lead to epiphora, growth in fundus, blepharitis and loss of eyelashes.

Majority of patients develop a hematopoietic disorder resembling Fanconi's anemia because initially the bone marrow is normal but gradually fat cells and fibrotic tissue replace the hematopoietic cells. Hematopoietic disorder manifests as marrow hypoplasia, anemia or thrombocytopenia. With development of pan-cytopenia, there occurs a secondary infection that is the cause of death in majority of these patients. In addition to marrow failure and malignant changes in white patches, pulmonary complications are also serious complications in patients with DC.

Immunologic abnormalities occur affecting both the humoral and cell-mediated immunity causing high incidence of opportunistic infections.

An abnormality in cell-mediated immunity is evident by delayed hypersensitivity reaction to skin test (antigen inoculation) and no sensitization to dinitrochlorobenzene. Abnormalities in immune systems like lymphoid depletion, absence of primary germinal follicles and fibrosis of lymph nodes can also occur.

There may be hyperpigmentation of the buccal mucosa that may be reactive postinflammatory hypermelanosis. Other abnormalities like alopecia, taurodontism, mental retardation, small genitals premature aging, nutmeg liver, horseshoe kidneys, amyloidosis and development of Hodgkin's disease and adenocarcinoma are also reported.

ORAL MANIFESTATIONS

In DC both the hard and the soft tissues in the oral cavity are affected. Oral mucosal changes manifests in the form of a white keratotic patch. Earlier cases reported of vesicles and ulcerations preceding development of leukoplakia. But these may represent herpetic infections which may occur due to immunocompromised status of these patients secondary to bone marrow suppression.

Intraorally, the white patch may affect the buccal mucosa, tongue (Fig. 15.4) or palate, with tongue most commonly affected as seen in our patient. Usually, white patch associated with dyskeratosis congenita is leukoplakia but lichen planus or lichenoid lesions instead of leukoplakia are also reported.

Lichenoid lesions may be a component of chronic graft-versus-host disease. Electron microscopy studies revealed that cells in dyskeratosis congenita have an embryonic immature nucleus, which have higher chances to undergo malignant transformation. In addition, barrier zone

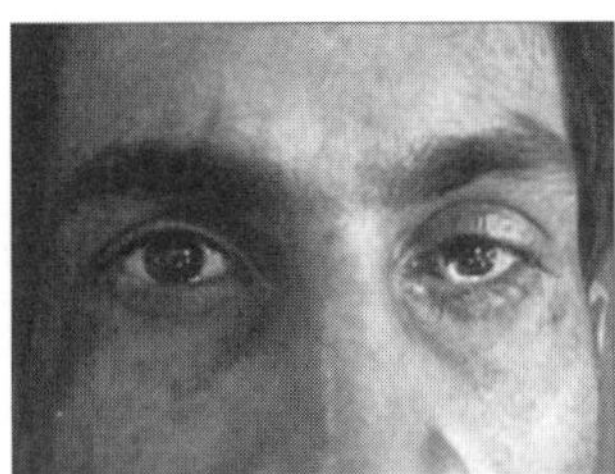

Fig. 15.1: Melanin pigmentation on the eye

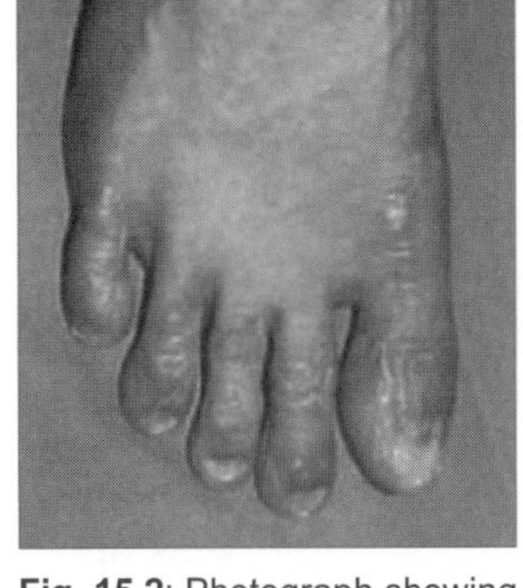

Fig. 15.2: Photograph showing cracking and missing nails of the toe

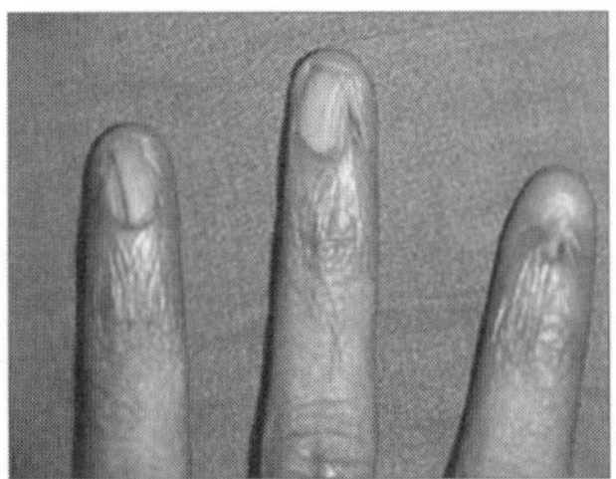

Fig. 15.3: Photograph showing cracking and missing nails of the hand

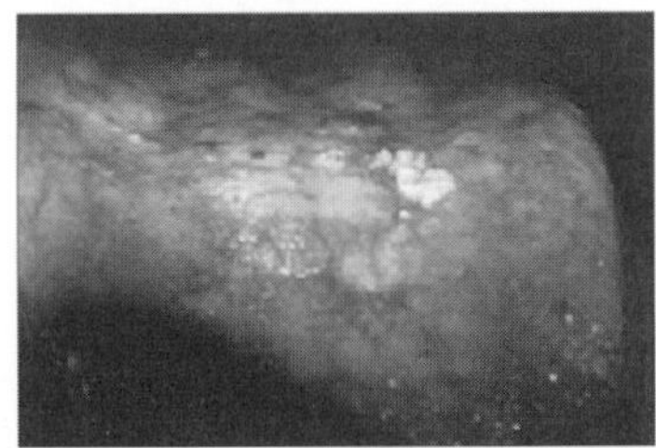

Fig. 15.4: Intraoral photograph showing a white patch on the dorsum of the tongue

of epithelium is less effective in dyskeratosis congenita than the normal epithelium causing increased permeability of noxious substances and carcinogens to the germinal layers. Hence increased malignant transformation rate is seen in leukoplakic areas associated with dyskeratosis congenita.

In DC severe periodontal destruction occur due to anomalies in ectodermally derived structures and diminished host response caused by neutropenia. Patients have gingival inflammation, bleeding, recession and bone loss that simulates juvenile periodontitis. In addition, there may be defects in the structure of the enamel like hypocalcification that may cause dental caries (Table 15.1).

Table 15.1: Oral findings in dyskeratosis congetina

Complications	*Manifestations*	*Etiology*
Infections	Dental caries, periodontitis and oral ulcerations	Defects in enamel, ectodermal structures and neutropenia
Hematologic	Bleeding and atrophic glossitis	Thrombocytopenia and anemia due to bone marrow suppression

Contd...

Contd...

Complications	*Manifestations*	*Etiology*
Oral mucosa	Leukoplakia, lichenoid lesions, pigmentation	Genetic, Graft Versus Host Disease (GVHD) and post-inflammatory pigmentation
Tooth Related		
a) In longitudinal ground sections	Thin enamel, indistinct incremental lines of Retzius, scanty enamel spindles, short enamel tufts, absence of gnarled enamel, abundance of enamel lamellae and flat interface between enamel and dentine	Defects in the ectodermal and ectomesenchymal derivatives
b) Clinical observations	Hypodontia, delayed eruption and short blunted roots	

HISTOLOGIC FINDINGS

Skin biopsy specimens from the areas of reticulated pigmentation typically show mild hyperkeratosis, epidermal atrophy, telangiectasia, epidermal atrophy, melanophages in the papillary dermis. Interface changes have also been reported, with mild basal layer vacuolization and a lymphocytic inflammatory infiltrate in the upper dermis. Oral lesions have not been thoroughly studied but the leukoplakic lesions appear to be nonspecific hyperparakeratosis or hyperorthokeratosis and acanthosis. Depending on the stage of the disease, the epithelium may show dysplasia.[2]

Differential Diagnosis

The differential diagnosis includes Fanconi's anemia, pachyonychia congenita, white spongy nevus and graft-versus-host disease (GVHD). DC is considered as a variant of Fanconi's anemia because aplastic anemia and cutaneous pigmentation occur in both but the 2 conditions differ from each other. Fanconi's anemia may have a possible association with oral squamous cell carcinoma. In contrast to dyskeratosis congenita, Fanconi's anemia is an autosomal dominant condition with concomitant skeletal and renal abnormalities. But there is no nail dystrophy or oral leukoplakia seen in Fanconi's anemia as reported in this case.[1]

Pachyonychia congenita is an autosomal dominant condition characterized by nail abnormalities, hyperkeratosis or hyperhidrosis of the palms and the sole and mucosal leukoplakia. In pachyonychia congenita, the nails become thick and shed at an early age and the mucosal leukoplakias do not undergo malignant transformation. Hematological abnormalities do not occur in pachyonychia congenita. White spongy nevus is a congenital leukokeratosis that presents with diffuse milky-white plaques on oral mucous membrane. The keratotic plaques are extensive and persist throughout life, without a tendency for malignant transformation. It is not associated with skin, nail or hematological abnormalities as seen in DC.

In patients with DC who have undergone bone marrow transplantation, graft-versus-host disease can be considered as a differential diagnosis because they have several features in common, including skin and nail changes. DC should be suspected in cases where the chronological pattern is not consistent with chronic graft-versus-host disease. In DC leukoplakias rather than lichenoid lesions occur. If white lesion shows lichenoid lesion like characteristics GVHD should be suspected.

TREATMENT

The discomfort of the oral lesions is managed symptomatically, and careful periodic oral mucosal examination is performed to check for evidence of malignant transformation. Routine medical evaluation is warranted to monitor the patient for the development of aplastic anemia. Selected patients may be considered for allogeneic bone marrow transplantation once the aplastic anemia is identified.

As a result of these potentially life-threatening complications, the prognosis is guarded. The average life span for the more severely affected patients is 32 years of age. The parents and the patients should receive genetic counseling, but identification of the DKC1 gene should allow for accurate confirmation of carriers of the gene and prenatal diagnosis.[3]

REFERENCES

1. Auluck A. Dyskeratosis congenita Dyskeratosis congenita. Report of a case with literature review; Med Oral Patol Oral Cir Bucal 2007;12:E369–73.
2. Shafer, Hine, Levy Textbook of Oral Pathology, 5th ed.
3. Neville, Damm, Allen, Bouquot. Oral and Maxillofacial Pathology, 2nd ed. Dermatologic diseases.

CHAPTER 16

White Sponge Nevus

(**Synonyms**: Familial white folded dysplasia of mucous membrane, white folded gingivostomatitis, oral epithelial nevus, congenital leukokeratosis, Cannon's disease)

INTRODUCTION

White sponge nevus (WSN) is a rare autosomal dominant disorder which was first described by Hyde in 1909, but the term was coined in 1935 by Cannon. It was also named as *familial white folded dysplasia.* The condition predominantly affects noncornifying stratified squamous epithelia, such as the oral mucosa and less frequently, extraoral sites, including the mucosal membrane of the nose, esophagus, rectum and vulvovaginal mucosa but not the skin.[1]

PATHOGENESIS

White sponge nevus is a relatively rare genodermatosis (a genetically determined skin disorder) that is inherited as an autosomal dominant trait displaying a high degree of penetrance and variable expressivity. This condition is due to a defect in the normal keratinization of the oral mucosa. In the 30-member family of keratin filaments, the pair of keratins known as keratin 4 and keratin 13 is specifically expressed in the spinous cell layer of mucosal epithelium. Mutations in either of these keratin genes have been shown to be responsible for the clinical manifestations of white sponge nevus.[3]

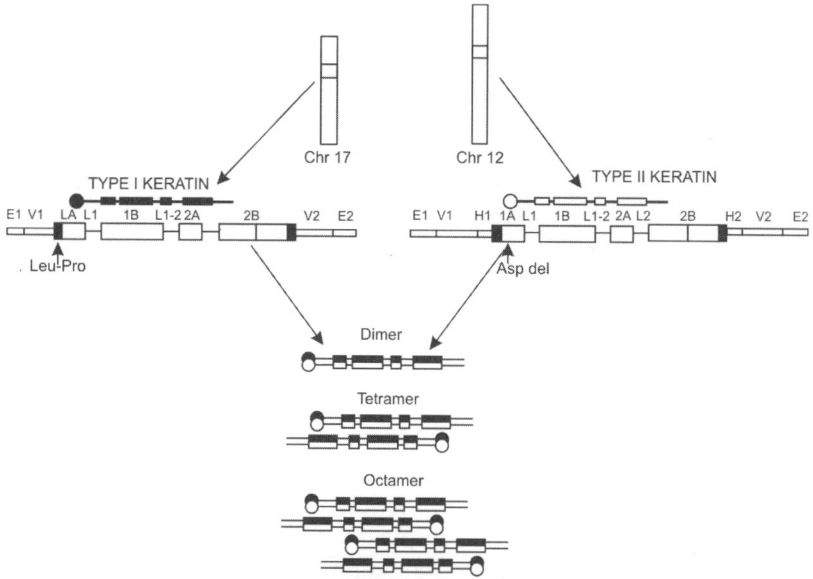

Flowchart 16.1: Pathogenesis of white sponge nevus

Representation of the type I and type II keratins and one of the possible ways of polymerization. The large white boxes represent the alpha-helical rod domain (1A, 1B, 2A, 2B) interrupted by short, nonhelical linker segments (L1, L1-2). The thinner boxes represent the nonhelical head and tail domains (E1, V1, E2, V2 and H1 in type II only). The arrows represent the approximate site of the mutation found on the keratin gene in WSN patients by Richard, et al. on K13 (Leu –> Pro; left panel) and by Rugg, et al. on K4 (Asp del; right panel). Both defects result in an abnormal K4/K13 heterodimer formation with irregular intermediate keratin filament fibers.[2] (Flowchart 16.1)

CLINICAL FEATURES AND ORAL MANIFESTATIONS

The lesions of white sponge nevus usually appear at birth or in early childhood, but sometimes the condition develops during adolescence. Clinically, white sponge nevus of the oral cavity is characterized by the presence of asymptomatic, bilateral, soft, white and spongy plaques. The surface of the plaque is thick, folded and may peel away from the underlying tissue. Lesions are asymptomatic and rough to palpation. The condition may involve the entire oral mucosa as to leave little normal mucosa visible, or may be distributed unilaterally as discrete white patches. The buccal mucosa (Fig. 16.1) is the most commonly affected site, followed by the soft palate, ventral tongue (Fig. 16.2), labial mucosa (Fig. 16.3), the alveolar ridges and the floor of the mouth. Gingival margin and dorsal aspect of tongue are usually spared. The disease is characterized by a wide variability and high penetrance, but with a benign clinical course. The size of lesions varies from patient to patient and time to time.

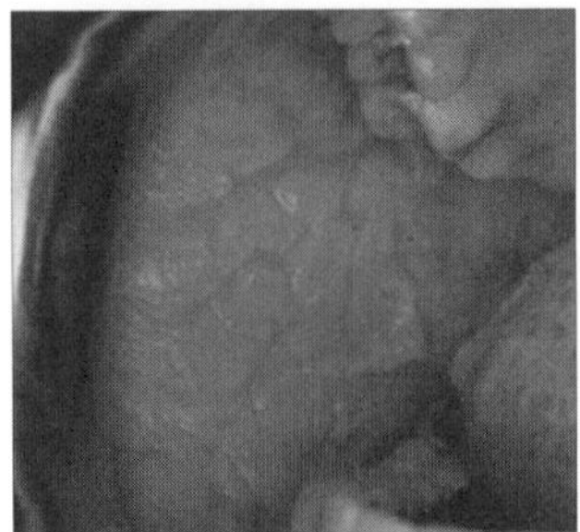

Fig. 16.1: Light rose fissured plaques of buccal mucosa

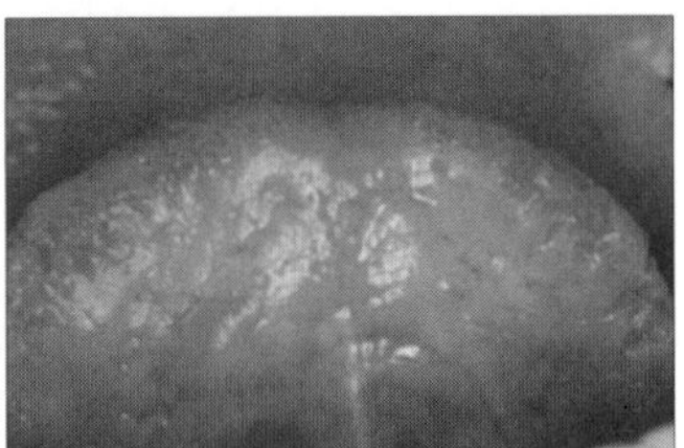

Fig. 16.2: Light rose spongy plaques of the tongue

HISTOLOGIC FEATURES

The microscopic features of white sponge nevus are characteristic but not necessarily pathognomonic. Prominent hyperparakeratosis and marked acanthosis with clearing of the cytoplasm of the cells in the spinous layer are common features (Fig. 16.4).[3] Parakeratotic plugs may extend into the prickle cells, giving a so-called basket weave appearance to the epithelium (Fig. 16.5). The underlying connective tissue is unremarkable.[2] However, similar microscopic findings may be associated with leukoedema and hereditary benign intraepithelial dyskeratosis (HBID). In some instances, an eosinophilic condensation is noted in the perinuclear region of the cells in the superficial layers of the epithelium (Fig. 16.6), a feature that is unique to white sponge nevus. Ultrastructurally, this condensed material can be identified as tangled masses of keratin tonofilaments.[3]

Exfoliative cytologic studies may provide more definitive diagnostic information. A cytologic preparation stained with the Papanicolaou method often shows the eosinophilic perinuclear condensation of the

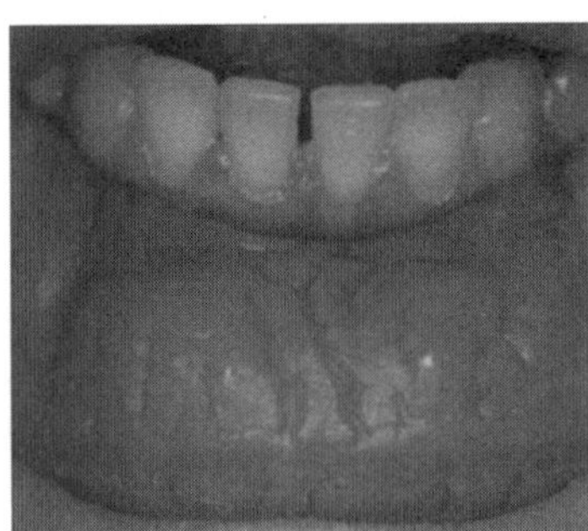

Fig. 16.3: Light rose fissured plaques of labial mucosa

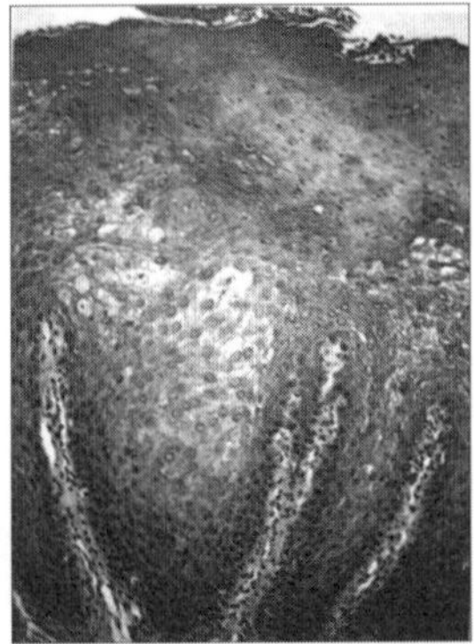

Fig. 16.4: Hematoxylin and eosin-stained section obtained from the buccal mucosa shows prominent parakeratosis, marked thickening (acanthosis), and vacuolation of the spinous cell layer

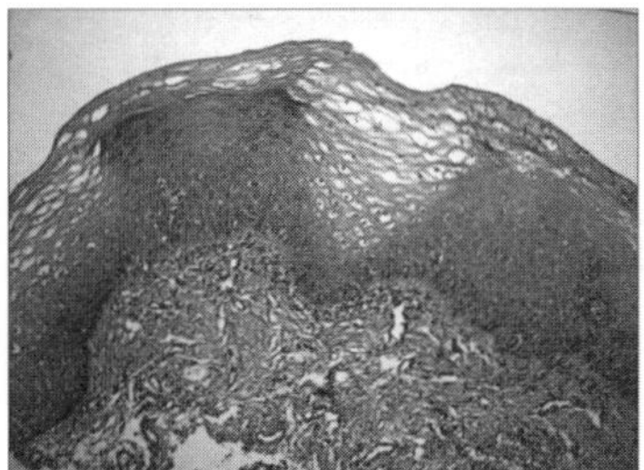

Fig. 16.5: H and E stained section showing a "basket weave" pattern within the epithelium. Basal cells appear normal

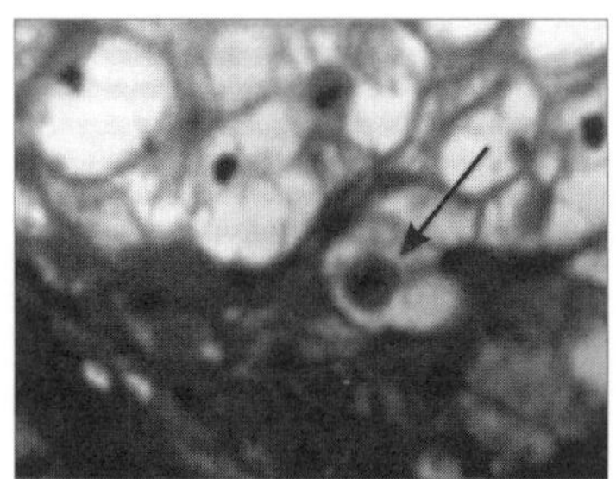

Fig. 16.6: High power section shows vacuolation of the cells of the spinous layer, with no evidence of epithelial atypia. Perinuclear condensation of keratin tonofilaments can be observed in some cells (arrow)

epithelial cell cytoplasm to a greater extent than does the histopathologic section (Fig. 16.7).

Diagnosis

The recognition of this disorder is important in that it must be differentiated from other congenital or familial disorders of more widespread clinical significance. The clinical appearance is so distinctive that biopsy is usually unnecessary. The diagnosis is made more certain if there is a positive family history and other mucous membranes are affected. In case of any suspicion, biopsy should be performed. The differential diagnosis of white sponge nevus includes oral lesions of leukoplakia, chemical burns, trauma, syphilis, tobacco and betel nut use. White sponge nevus may also be confused with candidiasis, but fungal examination, the histology of biopsy specimens, and the response to antifungal agents will be the differentiating factors. Cheek-biting, lichen planus, lupus erythematosus should also be excluded.

Lesions of pachyonychia congenita, hereditary benign intraepithelial dyskeratosis, Darier's disease, dyskeratosis congenita may resemble lesions of white sponge nevus. Except for lichen planus and lupus erythematosus which may be limited to the oral cavity, these disorders can be distinguished clinically from white sponge nevus by their associated extraoral lesions. Thus, concurrent skin lesions exclude the diagnosis of white sponge nevus. The histopathology of these conditions also varies.

TREATMENT

Although the patients suffer from no pain, they often complain of an altered texture of the mucosa or that the lesions are unaesthetic. Reassurance is all that is required, although numerous therapy models have been tried. None are likely to be effective unless they take into account the genetic nature of the lesions.

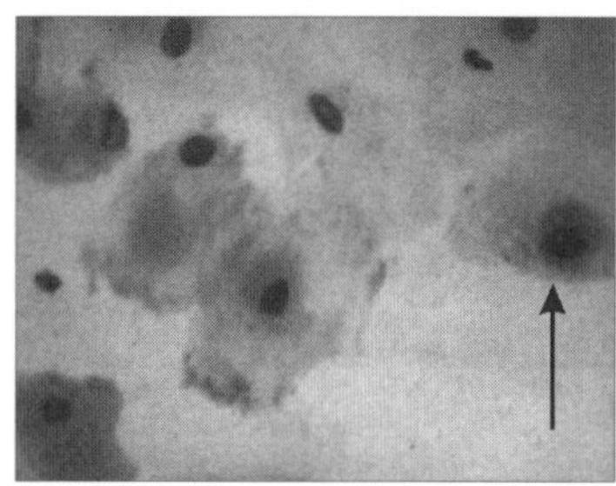

Fig. 16.7: High power section of Papanicolaou-stained cytologic preparation shows the pathognomonic perinuclear condensation of keratin tonofilaments (arrow)

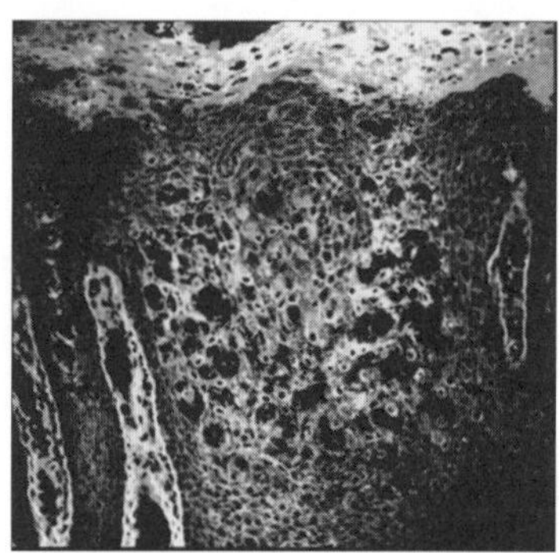

Fig. 16.8: Confocal laser scanner microscopy of the previous hematoxylin and eosin (H and E)-stained section: The spinous cell had enlarged with intracellular edema the clear cell keratinocytes were located from suprabasal to spinous layer

Treatment with vitamins, antihistaminics and mouth rinses have been recommended, but none has been successful. Penicillin was reported to succeed to a little extent in the management of WSN. Treatment in the form of gene therapy is difficult for a group of disorders including WSN due to autosomal dominant inheritance and the mutations acting in a dominant negative-manner. To achieve this the ways of inactivating mutant gene are actively being studied.

REFERENCES

1. European Association of Oral Medicine.
2. Gènes et peau. Euro J of Dermatol. Number 6, September 1997;405–8.
3. Neville, Damm, Allen, Bouquot. Oral and Maxillofacial Pathology, 2nd ed. Dermatologic Diseases.

CHAPTER

17

Warty Dyskeratosis

(**Synonyms**: Isolated Darier's disease, isolated dyskeratosis follicularis, focal acantholytic dyskeratosis)

INTRODUCTION[1]

The warty dyskeratoma is a distinctly uncommon solitary lesion that can occur on skin or oral mucosa. It is histopathologically identical to Darier's disease. For this reason, the lesion has been termed isolated Darier's disease. The lesion is not otherwise related to Darier's disease, however, and its cause remains unknown.

CLINICAL FEATURES

The cutaneous warty dyskeratoma typically appears as a solitary, asymptomatic, umblicated papule on the skin of the head or neck of an older adult. The intraoral lesion also develops in patients older than age 40, and a slight male predilection has been identified. The intraoral warty dyskeratoma appears as a pink or white, umblicated papule located on the keratinized mucosa, specially the hard palate and the alveolar ridge. A warty or roughened surface is noted in some lesions. Most warty dyskeratomas are smaller than 0.5 cm in diameter.

HISTOLOGIC FEATURES[2]

Histolopathologically, the warty dyskeratoma appears very similar to keratosis follicularis. Both conditions display dyskeratosis and a suprabasilar cleft. The warty dyskeratoma is a solitary lesion, however, and the formation of corps ronds and grains is not a prominent feature.

TREATMENT AND PROGNOSIS

Treatment of the warty dyskeratoma consists of conservative excision. The prognosis is excellent; these lesions have not been reported to recur, and they have no evaluation of the tissue should be performed because some epithelial dysplasias may show a marked lack of cellular cohesiveness, resulting in a similar acantholytic appearance microscopically.

REFERENCES

1. Shafer-Hine–Levy Textbook of Oral Pathology, 5th ed.
2. Neville, Damm, Allen, Bouquot. Oral and Maxillofacial Pathology, 2nd ed. Dermatologic Diseases.

CHAPTER 18

Cowden Syndrome

(**Synonym**: Multiple hamartoma syndrome)

INTRODUCTION

Cowden syndrome was first described by Lloyd and Dennis in 1963 referring to their patient Rachael Cowden, who died of breast carcinoma. Weary and coworkers reported a further 5 patients in 1972 and suggested the name multiple hamartoma syndrome (MHS).[2]

Cowden syndrome is an infrequent genodermatosis clinically expressede in the skin, mucosas and multiple organs, with an autosomal dominant-inheritance pattern, of incomplete penetration and variable expressivity. It is part of the diseases known as "hamartosis" due to the presence of multiple hamartomas originated in any of the three embryonic layers. Some of the lesions are prone to malignization, therefore, the disease belongs to the "preneoplastic hereditary syndromes".[1]

PATHOGENESIS

The etiology is unknown, although since 1993 it has been related with the presence of alterations in the phosphatase and tensin homologue (PTEN) gene, on the long arm of chromosome 10 (10q23.31, 10q22.3) or mutated in multiple advanced cancers (MMAC1), this normally acts as a tumor suppressor gene and on occasions is mutated in breast, prostate and brain tumors.[2]

CLINICAL FEATURES[3]

The prevalence of Cowden syndrome is 1:200,000 making it what is considered to be a rare disease. Cowden syndrome shows multiple hamartomas of endodermic, ectodermic or mesodermic origin. Despite being treated as a disease within the gastrointestinal area, its extraintestinal clinical manifestations are manifest and on numerous occasions determine the patient's prognosis.

Gastrointestinal Manifestations

Manifestations of Cowden syndrome in the gastrointestinal tract are practically indistinguishable from family juvenile polyposis syndrome. They are characterized by the presence of multiple hamartomatous polyps along the gastrointestinal tract, principally located in the colon and rectum, generally asymptomatic, a fact that contributes to the underdiagnosis of the disease. Histologically they are characterized by presenting a high number of normotypical glands of mucoid content, inflammation and edema of the lamina propria and lymphoplasmocytic infiltration. We may also find ganglioneuromas and lipomatous and inflammatory polyps and ganglioneuromas. In the esophagus, it is possible to find glycogenic acanthosis without associated clinical repercussions.

Extraintestinal Manifestations

Unlike with other polyposis, systemic manifestations of Cowden syndrome are abundant and sufficiently distinctive, which can determine their clinical diagnosis. Mucocutaneous lesions are the most notable manifestations of Cowden syndrome; in fact approximately 80% of patients diagnosed with the syndrome of multiple hamartomas has or will develop some manifestation of this type in the future.

These are usually lesions that evolve over a long period of time and which, generally speaking, manifest themselves in the initial stages, before the other neoplastic processes associated with the disease develop, which shows the importance of detecting these benign lesions early and beginning adequate tumoral screening for early diagnosis. The most notable types of these lesions are facial trichilemmomas, acral keratosis, subcutaneous lipomas, palmoplantar keratosis, oral and labial papillomas with a characteristic cobbled look. The appearance of vitiligo, neuromas, xanthomas and café-au-lait spots is less commonly associated with Cowden syndrome (Fig. 18.1).

Although these are the most noted clinical manifestations, these lesions can be accompanied by otorhinolaryngological, ophthalmological, gynecological, renal and craniomaxillofacial manifestations. Because of its special importance, it is imperative to underscore the high risk associated with developing neoplastic pathologies, mainly of the breast and thyroid, without overlooking the possibility of developing other types of neoplasia (ovarian, uterus, kidney and meninx).

Oral Manifestations[4]

The oral lesions vary in severity from patient to patient and usually consist of multiple papules affecting the gingivae, dorsal tongue, and buccal mucosa. These lesions have been reported in more than 80% of affected patients and generally produce no symptoms. Other possible oral findings include high arched palate, periodontitis, and extensive dental caries, although it is unclear whether the latter two conditions are significantly related to the syndrome (Figs 18.2 to 18.5).

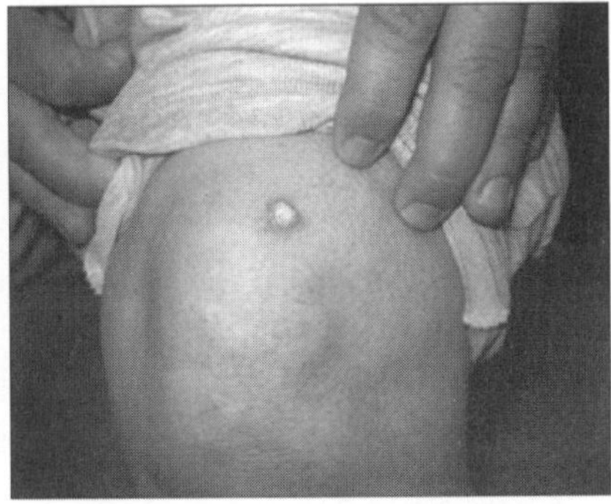

Fig. 18.1: Cutaneous trichilemmomas in acral regions

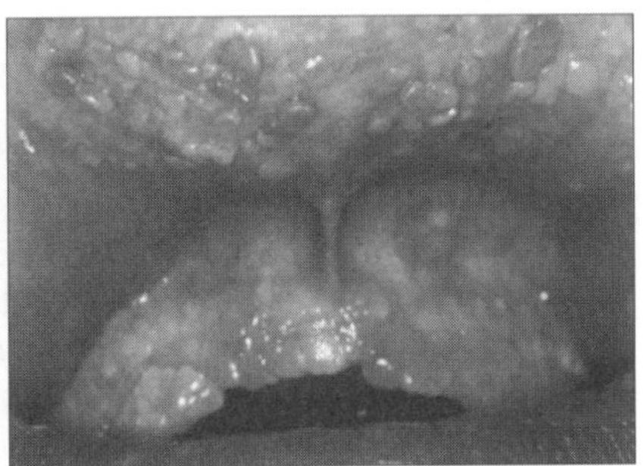

Fig. 18.2: Multiple papules on the gingiva, upper and lower lip. Aspect similar to small "round stones"

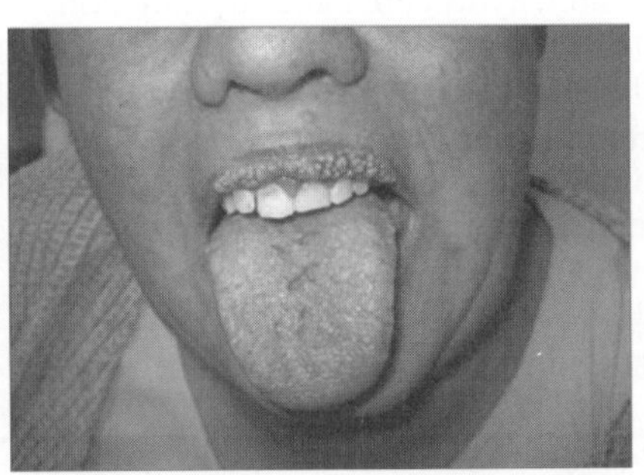

Fig. 18.3: Multiple lesions of a papillomatous lesions on upper lip with scrotal tongue

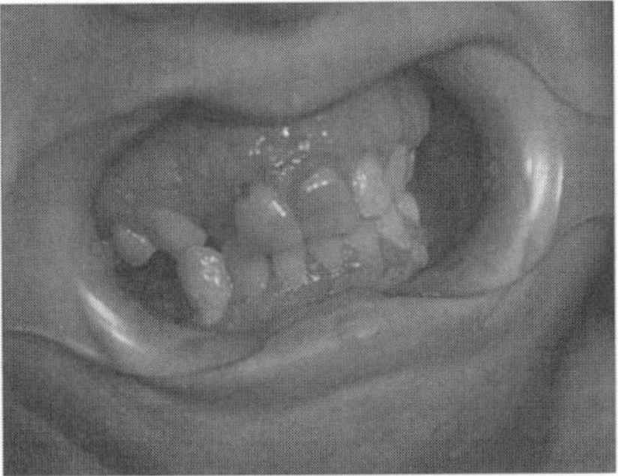

Fig. 18.4: Numerous papules on the gingiva giving rise to a cobblestone appearance

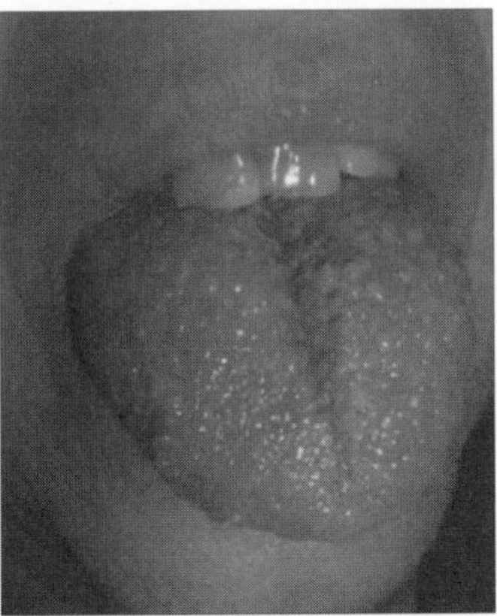

Fig. 18.5: Moriform appearance of the tongue due to the enormous amount of papules

Oral fibromas present as smooth whitish-pink papules on the mucosa of the oral cavity, when arranged in groups they give rise to a typical cobblestone image.

Summary of main clinical findings of Cowden syndrome[2]

Location	*Abnormality*
Mucocutaneous	Multiple facial trichilemmomas, oral papillomas, actinic keratosis lymphomas, vitiligo
Thyroid gland	Goiter, adenomas, adenocarcinomas, thyroiditis, hyper and hypothyroidism, cysts of thyroglossal duct
Breast	Fibrocystic disease, carcinoma, intraductal papilloma, atypical ductal hyperplasia
Gastrointestinal	Polips of various types, including adenomatous, hamartomatous, lipomatous, lymphomatous, hyperplastic, and diverticulum of the colon
Central nervous system	Ganglionic neurons, neurofibromas, intracranial hypertension, hydrocephalous, dysfunction of cerebella and cranial nerves, subarachnoid hemorrhage, meningioma
Genitourinary	*Female*—Irregular periods, ovarian cysts, leiomyomas, teratomas, uterine fibroma, adenocarcinoma of the urethra, cervix and kidney, vaginal cysts *Male*—Hydrocele, varicocele, hypoplastic testicles
Skeletal	Increased cranium size, kyphosis, kyphoscoliosis, pectus Excavatum, large hands and feet, syndactyly, mandibular and maxillary hypoplasia
Visual	Hypertelorism, congenital vascular abnormalities, glaucoma, myopia
Cardiovascular	Hypertension, prolapse of mitral valve, aortic insufficiency
Respiratory	Polips of the larynx, pulmonary cysts, bilateral pulmonary lipomatosis

Histologic Features

The histopathologic features of the oral lesions are rather nonspecific, essentially representing fibroepithelial hyperplasia. Other lesions associated with this syndrome have their own characteristic histopathologic findings, depending on the hamartomatous or neoplastic tissue origin (Fig. 18.6).[4]

Diagnosis[3]

Diagnosis is mainly based on clinical criteria. At this time the diagnostic method of major and minor clinical criteria proposed by Salem and Steck

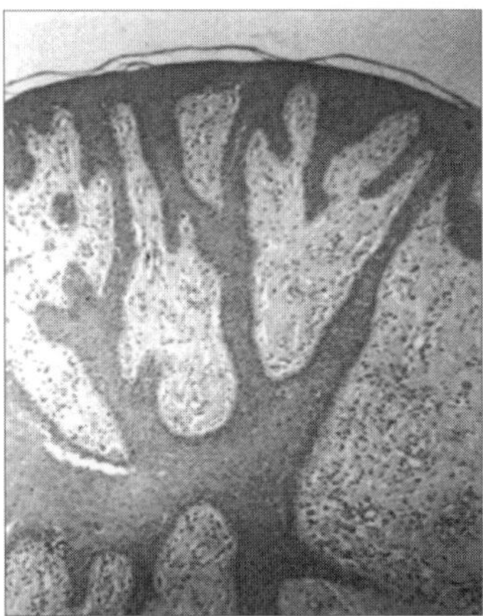

Fig. 18.6: Histopathologic picture (H and E) of papillary-like epithelial hyperplasia of the oral mucosa

as subsequently revised and modified by the International Cowden Consortium in 2000 is the accepted one (Table 18.1). Cowden syndrome is diagnosed when the patient shows one of the following criteria:

1. Presence of pathognomonic lesions, always when under one of the following conditions:
   - Six or more facial papules, of which three or more must be trichilemmomas.
   - Facial papules and papillomatosis in oral mucosa.
   - Papillomatosis in oral mucous and acral keratosis.
   - Six or more palmoplantar keratosis lesions.
2. Presence of 2 major criteria, one of which must be macrocephalia or Lhermitte-Duclos disease.
3. Presence of 1 major criterion and 3 minor criteria.
4. Presence of 4 minor criteria.

Table 18.1: Pathognomonic lesions and major and minor criteria

Pathognomonic lesions	*Major criteria*	*Minor criteria*
Fascial trichilemmomas Acral keratosis Papillomatous papules Mucous lesions	Mammary carcinoma Thyroid carcinoma (mainly follicular) Macrocephalia Lhermitte-Duclos disease Endometrial carcinoma	Other thyroid pathology Mental retardation Intestinal hamartomatous polyps Fibrocystic mammary disease Lipomas Fibromas Urogenital tumors Urogenital malformations

Cowden syndrome can be diagnosed for a direct relative of an affected patient if he or she meets one of the following conditions:

1. Mucocutaneous pathognomonic lesions
2. Any major criterion with or without associated minor criteria
3. Presence of 2 minor criteria.

DIFFERENTIAL DIAGNOSIS[2]

It is important to make a correct differential diagnosis of the fibropapillomatosis lesions of oral mucosa such as multiple pointed condyloma, multiple traumatic fibromas, multiple neuromas, acanthosis nigricans, Darier disease, Heck's disease, phenytoin hyperplasia, tuberous sclerosis, lymphangioma, pyogenic granuloma, epidermoid or squamous carcinoma.

TREATMENT

Treatment of multiple hamartoma syndrome is controversial. Although most of the tumors that develop are benign, the prevalence of malignancy is higher than in the general population. Some investigators recommend bilateral prophylactic mastectomies as early as the third decade of life for female patients because of the associated increased risk of breast cancer.

REFERENCES

1. Blanco V, Keochgerián V. Cowden's syndrome. Case report with reference to an affected family. Med Oral Patol Oral Cir Bucal 2006;1:E12–6.
2. Jair C. Leão, a Virgínia Batista Cowden's syndrome affecting the mouth, gastrointestinal, and central nervous system: A case report and review of the literature. Oral Surg Oral Med Oral Pathol Oral Radiol Endod 2005;99: 569–72.
3. Cañadas LMC, Sánchez JLS. Multiple oral fibropapillomatosis as an initial manifestation of cowden syndrome. Case report. Med Oral Patol Oral Cir Bucal 2006;11:E319–24.
4. Neville, Damm, Allen, Bouquot. Oral and maxillofacial pathology, 2nd ed. Dermatologic Diseases.

CHAPTER

19

Peutz-Jeghers Syndrome

(**Synonyms**: Hereditary intestinal polyposis syndrome, intestinal hamartous polyps in association with mucocutaneous melanocytic macules)

INTRODUCTION

Peutz-Jeghers syndrome (PJS) is rare syndrome that was first described by Y Peutz, a Dutch pediatrician, in 1921 a family with skin pigmentation and polyps of the small bowel. Similar cases were reported in US by H Jeghers and colleagues in 1949 and consequently the name of Peutz-Jeghers syndrome (PJS) was adopted for this disorder. PJS is an inherited, autosomal dominant disorder characterized by mucocutaneous pigmentation and gastrointestinal polyps. Melanic spots are the earliest manifestation of PJS, typically appearing in the first year of life. Although most of the polyps reside in the jejunum, it may also occur in ileum, stomach, duodenum and/or colon. Those polyps are present from childhood and may sometimes lead to intussusception or gastrointestinal bleeding.[1]

PATHOGENESIS

PJS is an autosomal dominant inherited syndrome. The cause of the syndrome appears to be a germline mutation of the gene STK11 (also know as LKB1) located at 19p13.3. Germline mutation of STK11 are documented in upto 70–80% of patients with PJS and upto 15% of cases have deletions of all or part of STK11.[1]

The STK11 gene is a tumor suppressor gene that encodes a serine-threonine kinase that modulates cellular proliferation, controls cell polarity, and seems to have an important role in responding to low cellular energy levels.[1]

To exert this last role, the STK11 protein is involved in the inhibition of AMP-activated protein kinase (AMPK), and signals downstream to inhibit the mTOR (mammalian target of rapamycin; also known as FRAP; FKBP12—rapamycin complex-associated protein) pathway. The mTOR pathway seems disregulated in patients with PJS.[1]

Genotype–phenotype correlation suggests that patients with PJS who have mutations in SKT 11 that result in truncation of the encoded STK11 protein have a significantly earlier age of onset than those who have missense mutation of detectable mutation of STK11.[1]

Apart from this the role of beta-cathenice, adenomatous polyposis coli, K-ras and p-53 gene mutations have also been investigated.[2]

CLINICAL FEATURES[1]

PJS is an autosomal dominant inherited syndrome consisting of gastro-intestinal hamartoma and mucocutaneous hyperpigmentation, having an estimated prevalence of 1 in 120000 live births without racial or sexual predilection.

The characteristic pigmentation is present in more than 90% of patients with PJS. The pigmented maculae may be present at birth but usually develop in early childhood, and even may develop later in life occasionally. Round, oval or irregular patches of brown or almost black pigmentation 1–5 mm in diameter are most commonly find around the mouth, nose, lower lip, buccal mucosa, hands and feet. Perianal and genital regions may also be involved. Oral pigmentation is usually permanent, but the maculae on the lips and skin may fade after puberty. Rarely, the nails may be pigmented, diffusely or in longitudinal bands (Fig. 19.1).

The pigmented maculae arise from increased number of melanocytes at the dermoepidermal junction, with increased melanin in basal cells. It should distinguish these melanin deposits from ordinary freckles. Freckles are absent at birth (but may occur in infancy) are sparse near the nostrils and mouth, and never appear on the oral mucosa (Figs 19.2 and 19.3).

Gastrointestinal polyps in PJS are hamartoma. Hamartomatous polyps are composed of the normal cellular elements of the gastrointestinal tract, but have a markedly distorted architecture.

The hamartomatous polyposis syndromes are a heterogeneous group of disorders inherited in an autosomal-dominant manner. Apart from PJS, these syndromes include juvenile polyposis syndromes and PTEN hamartoma tumor syndrome (PHTS). PHTS include Cowden syndrome,

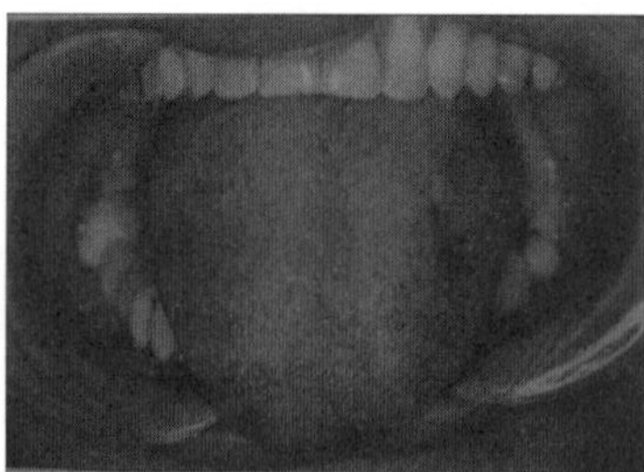

Fig. 19.1: Multiple perioral and oral mucosal melanotic macules are common in Peutz-Jegher's syndrome

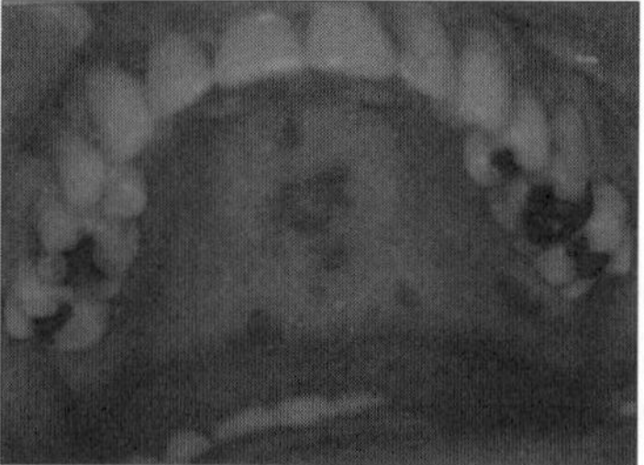

Fig. 19.2: Melanotic macules on palate

Bannayan-Riley-Ruvalcaba syndrome (BRRS), and all syndromes in which there are germline PTEN mutations.

The Peutz-Jeghers polyp is a unique hamartomatous lesion characterized by glandular epithelium that covers an arborizing framework of well-developed smooth muscle that is continuous with the muscularis mucosae. The smooth muscle band fan out into the head of the polyp and become progressively thinner as they project toward the surface of the polyp. Unlike the case of the juvenile polyp, the lamina propria is normal, and the characteristic architecture of the lesion appears to derive chiefly from the abnormal smooth muscle tissue.

These polyps are usually multiple and their distinctive appearance, in association with extraintestinal manifestations, makes PJS easily identifiable. The most common location for polyps is the small bowel (64%), although involvement of the colon (53%) stomach (49%) and rectum (32%) is also described.

Patients are diagnosed usually in the second or third decade of life and common presentations include abdominal pain, rectal bleeding, anemia, small intestinal intussusception, bowel obstruction, and rectal prolaps of polyps. Abdominal symptoms tend to occur early in life, with more than 50% symptomatic patients before the age of 20.

Histologic Features

The gastrointestinal polyps represent benign over growths of intestinal glandular epithelium supported by a core of smooth muscle. Epithelial atypia is not usually a prominent feature, unlike the polyps of Gardner syndrome.

Microscopic evaluation of the pigmented cutaneous lesions shows slight acanthosis of the epithelium with elongation of the rete ridges. No apparent increase in melanocyte number is detected by electron microscopy, but the dendritic processes of the melanocytes are elongated. Furthermore, the melanin pigment appears to be retained in the melanocytes rather than being transferred to adjacent keratinocytes.[3]

DIAGNOSIS

The diagnostic criteria for PJS include the presence of characteristic mucocutaneous pigmentation, small bowel hamartomatous polyps and family history of PJS. Patients need to fulfill two of these three criteria for the diagnosis.[1]

DIFFERENTIAL DIAGNOSIS

Normal variation vs syndrome or without polyposis is the most common differential.[4] In those individuals without intestinal polyposis, a familial history or sufficient numbers of melonotic macules in the common locations must be demonstrated for a diagnosis of PJS. This may be particularly difficult in blacks or other dark-skinned individuals who have melanotic oral macules normally. Addison disease is the other serious differential because of its oral and cutaneous macule hyperpigmentation. Although hereditary polyposis is known to occur in Gardner syndrome, juvenile polyposis and familial polyposis coli, none of these are associated with skin or oral melanotic macules and all have polyps limited to the colon. Albright syndrome and hereditary neurofibromatosis both manifest melanotic macular areas called *café-au-lait* macules. However, neither is associated with intestinal polyposis, and their melanotic macules are usually larger and found in areas other than the perioral, hand, perianal, and perigenital areas common to PJS (Fig. 19.4).

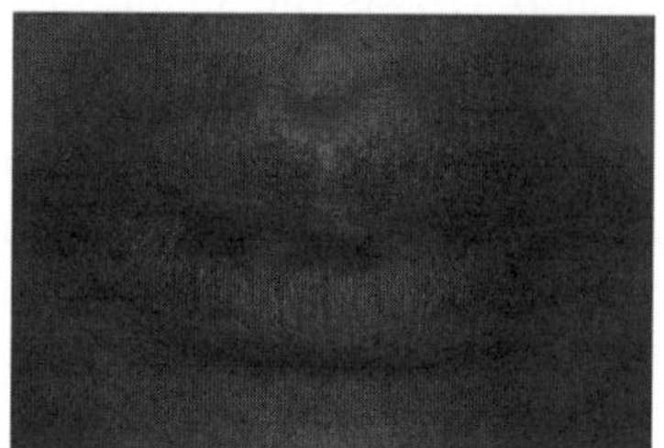

Fig. 19.3: Melanotic macules on lower lip vermillion

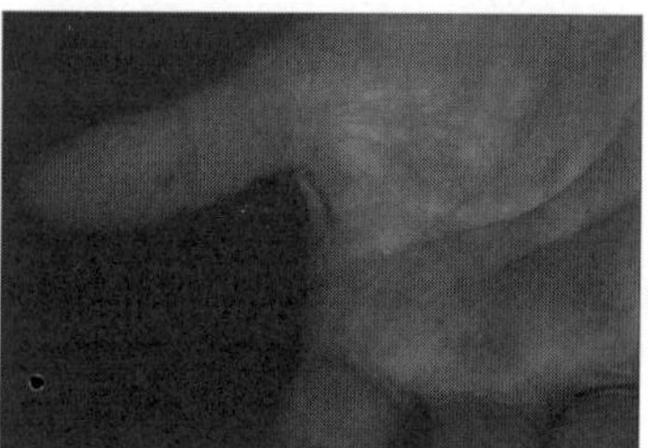

Fig. 19.4: Melanotic macules frequently seen on the hands

TREATMENT AND PROGNOSIS

Patients with Peutz-Jeghers should be monitored for development of intussusception or tumor formation, genetic counseling is also appropriate.

REFERENCES

1. Georgescu EF, Stanescu L, Peutz–Jeghers syndrome: Case report and literature review. Romanian Journal of Morphology and Embryology 2008;49(2):241–5.
2. Hacı Mehmet SÖKMEN Ali Tuzun NCE. A Peutz-Jeghers syndrome case with iron deficiency anemia and jejunojejunal invagination. Turk J Gastroenterol 2003;14(1):78–82.
3. Neville, Damm, Allen, Bouquot. Oral and Maxillofacial Pathology, 2nd ed. Dermatologic Diseases.
4. Marx. Oral and Maxillofacial Pathology.

CHAPTER 20
Hereditary Benign Intraepithelial Dyskeratosis

(**Synonym**: Witkop-Von Sallmann syndrome)

INTRODUCTION

Hereditary benign intraepithelial dyskeratosis (HBID) is a rare autosomal dominant hereditary genodermatosis first described in 1960 by Von Sallmann and Paton.[1] It was first noted in an isolated population of individuals in Halifax country, North Carolina, whose ancestors were a mix of African-heritage blacks, Native Americans, and Caucasian whites.

CLINICAL PRESENTATION

Hereditary benign intraepithelial dyskeratosis affects primarily oral and ocular mucosa with onset usually at birth or early childhood. Oral lesions are usually asymptomatic and may vary in extent. Most oral lesions go unrecognized until examined.[1]

Oral Manifestations

The oral mucosa is affected throughout, with the exception of the dorsum of the tongue, and develops wide areas of soft, spongy white lesions resembling clinical leukoplakia (Fig. 20.1). The buccal mucosal lesions are the most prominent and will often extend onto the commissure. As the individual matures, the lesions increase in area and often become folded and variegated in appearance between white and a translucent mucosal color.[2]

Ocular lesions in HBID begin early in life, being noted in nearly all affected persons by the age of 1 year. Eye lesions are typically bilateral[1] and appear as superficial, foamy, gelatinous plaques of the bulbar conjunctiva (i.e. the conjunctiva covering the globe) that form just outward from the limbus (the junction of the cornea and bulbar conjunctiva) (Figs 20.2A to D). These plaques are associated with conjunctival hyperemia, as noted by an increased number and size of vessels, but not a true conjunctivitis. There is no true inflammation.[2] When the lesions are active, patient may experience tearing, photophobia, and itching of the eyes. In many patients, the

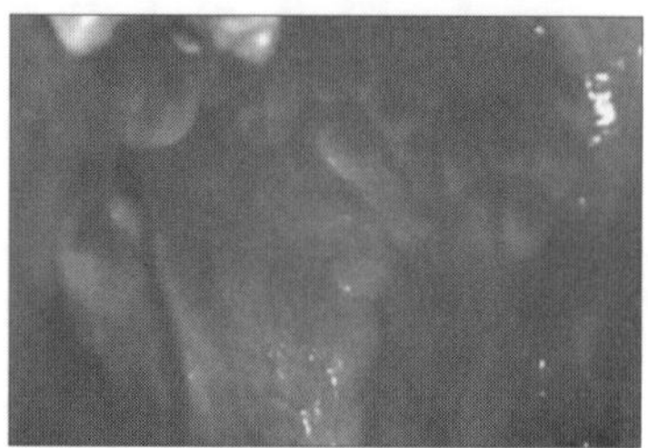

Fig. 20.1: Intraoral view demonstrating white diffuse rough plaques in the right buccal mucosa

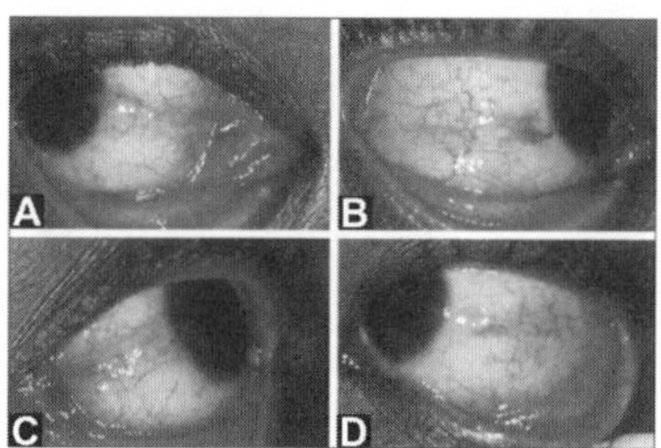

Figs 20.2A to D: Ocular bilateral gelatinous conjunctival plaques with dilated blood vessels. Internal (A) and external (B) aspects of the right eye, and in internal (C) and external (D) aspects of the left eye

plaques are most prominent in the spring and tend to regress during the summer or autumn. Sometimes blindness may result from the induction of vascularity of the cornea secondary to the shedding process.[3]

Histopathology

The histopathologic features of HBID include prominent parakeratin production in addition to marked acanthosis. A peculiar dyskeratotic process, similar to that of Darier's disease, is scattered throughout the upper spinous layer of the surface epithelium. With this dyskeratotic process, an epithelial cell appears to be surrounded or engulfed by an adjacent epithelial cell, resulting in the so-called "cell-within-a-cell" phenomenon.[3] (Figs 20.3A to C).

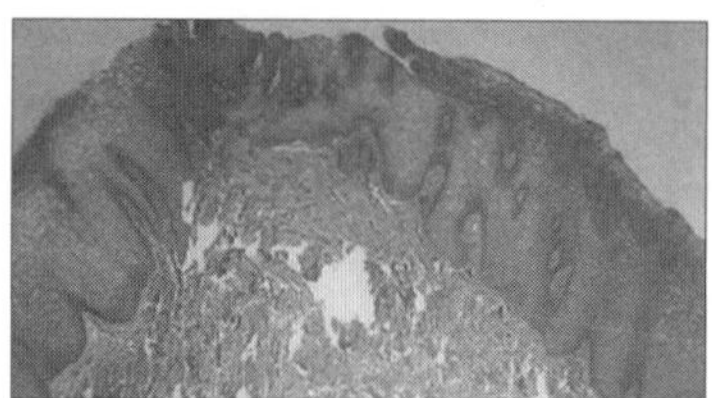

Fig. 20.3A: Epithelial thickness, hyperplasia, acanthosis, and vacuolated cells

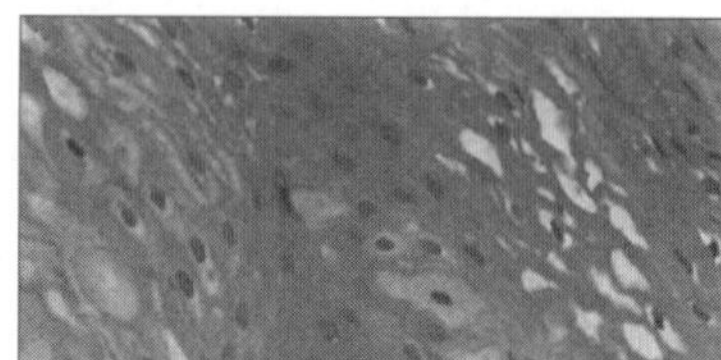

Fig. 20.3B: Dyskeratotic cells in the superficial layers

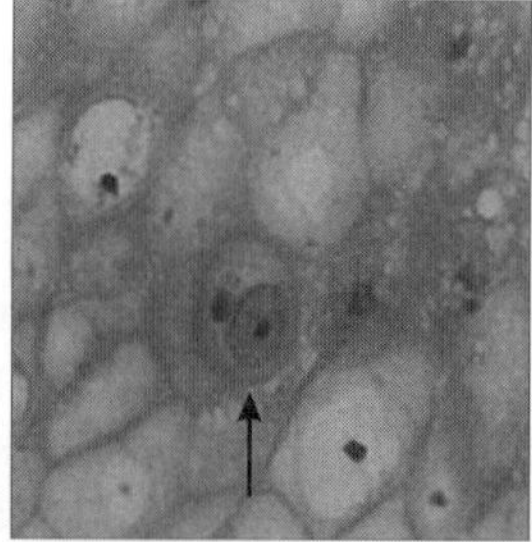

Fig. 20.3C: Engulfed cell (arrow), in a cell-within-cell pattern

Differential Diagnosis

The oral lesions are very similar to those seen in white sponge nevus, lichen planus, and the oral component of the two pachyonychia congenital variants, Jadassohn-Lewandowsky syndrome and Jackson-Lawler syndrome. However, neither white sponge nevus nor lichen planus produces conjunctival plaques as are seen in HBID. Lichen planus can produce a diffuse conjunctivitis at times, but not plaques. The pachyonychia congenita syndromes can be distinguished by their palmar and plantar hyperkeratosis as well as their prominent elevations of the toenails and fingernails. Benign nonspecific hyperkeratosis and even dysplastic or premalignant erythroleukoplakia may be considered in adult cases with mature HBID lesions. These lesions require a biopsy to distinguish them.

TREATMENT

Hereditary benign intraepithelial dyskeratosis is an entirely benign condition. Hence, no further treatment is required for oral lesions after establishment of diagnosis. Several modalities of treatment have been attempted for eye lesions, including topical medications and surgical procedures. However, the abnormal epithelium almost invariably recurs after excision.

REFERENCES

1. Jham BC, Mesquita RA, Aguiar MCF, Carmo MAV. Hereditary benign intraepithelial dyskeratosis: A new case? J Oral Pathol Med 2007;36:55–7.
2. Marx R. Oral and Maxillofacial Pathology.
3. Neville, Damm, Allen, Bouquot. Oral and Maxillofacial Pathology, 2nd ed. Dermatologic Diseases.

Index

A

Acantholysis 45
Acanthosis nigricans 107
Anti-Sm 92
Arthus reaction 20
Atrophy 6

B

Bulla 3

C

Café-au-lait macules 130
Calcinosis 36
Cobblestone mucosal 105
Collagen
  type IV 66
  type VII 66
Colloid, Civatte bodies 29
Corps ronds 106
Crust 4
Cyst 3

D

Disease
  Darier's 102, 119
  Graft-versus-host disease (GVHD) 112
  Graves' 18
  Hidebound 33

E

Ecchymoses 6
Erosion 5
Excoriation 5

F

Fissure 5

G

Genodermatosis 114

H

Hypohidrosis 11
Hypotrichosis 11

I

Iris or target 77

L

Laminin 5 epiligrin kalinin, uncein Laminin 6 66*f*
Langerhans cells 22
Libman-Sacks endocarditis 91
Lichenification 4
Lichenoid mucositis 25

M

Macule 2
Melanic spots 127
Milia 98
Morphea 35
Munro abscesses 43

N

Nodule 3

P

Pachyonychia congenita 112
Papule 2

Pemphigoid
- cicatricial 60
- ocular 60
- oral mucous membrane 60

Pemphigus 45
Pemphix 45
Petechiae 6
Photosensitivity 90
Plaque 2
Polyarteritis nodosa 20
Polyposis 128
Purpura 6
Pustule 4

R

Rash
- discoid 90
- malar butterfly 90

Raynaud's phenomenon 39

S

Scale 4
Scar 5
Sclerodactyly 38, 39
Scleroderma 33
SERCA2 102
Serum sickness 20
Sign 42, 51, 99
- Auspitz 42
- Nikolsky 51, 99

Syndrome
- Cowden 121
- CREST 39
- Goodpasture 19
- Lyell's 80
- Papillon-Lefevre 107
- Penogingival 26
- Peutz-Jeghers 127
- Stevens-Johnson 79
- vulvovaginal-gingival 26

T

Telangiectasia 7
Typical targets 75

U

Ulceration 5
Ulcers 6

V

Vesicle 3

W

Wheal 3
Wickham striae 27